30 DAYS
to UNDERSTANDING
CHRONIC ILLNESS
AND PAIN

CASEY CHAFFEY

Published by

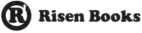 **Risen Books**

Richmond, Kentucky

2021

Printed by CreateSpace,
An Amazon.com Company

Published by Risen Books

ISBN-13: 978-0-9960087-7-8

Book design by Eric Dean,
ejdcreative.com

ENDORSEMENTS

"Casey Chaffey offers more than just a how-to guide for chronic pain and chronic illness sufferers. Readers will find plenty of helpful information in this short guide, but they will also encounter empathy from someone who understands what they are going through and hope for better care and treatment. While I don't deal with chronic pain or illness personally, I treat patients every day who do, and reading Casey's book has taught me to have more compassion for people with invisible illnesses. If you or someone you know has chronic pain or illness, this book is worth your time."

— STEVEN G., RN HOSPICE CASE MANAGER

"Facing life with chronic illness or pain can feel like being forced to move to a foreign country where everything is different and uncomfortable, you don't understand the lingo, and you're desperately homesick for your old way of life. Far from an exciting adventure, you can quickly become overwhelmed and lack the brain power to figure out how to cope with your limitations. Casey Chaffey is a gracious guide for your journey, coming alongside fellow sufferers with this easily-readable book. Each short chapter is packed with informative stats and definitions, practical ideas, and understanding encouragement. Caregivers and friends of the chronically ill will also find this a valuable read, as Casey gives an insightful peek into the mental and emotional burdens that are an inescapable part of daily life for those who can no longer trust their bodies. Perhaps most importantly, this book is a heartening reminder that you are not alone on this often-bewildering trek into the unknown: hope and help are here."

— Abigail W., adrenal fatigue, hormone imbalance, and scoliosis

"Casey Chaffey does an outstanding job articulating the struggles of living with chronic illness. In this book, she provides much needed validation to the tribulations we endure on a daily basis. Whether you are a patient or close to someone who has a chronic illness, this book is truly a must have. Even as someone who lives with many chronic conditions, I learned interesting things that I didn't know. The words made me feel heard and not alone. Thank you for providing such understandable content on a hard topic. I most definitely recommend *30 Days to Understanding Chronic Illness and Pain* as it's so easy and understandable to read."

— Rachael W., Ehlers Danlos Syndrome, POTS, adrenal insufficiency, spinal instability, tethered cord, intracranial hypertension

ACKNOWLEDGEMENTS

It takes more than an author to turn information into a published work, and this book would not exist without all the people behind the scenes. Thank you to my family who encouraged me in this endeavor and helped me along the way. Thank you to Steve for taking the time to edit and Eric for the amazing illustrations and cover design. Thank you to the readers. I hope this book in some small way helps to spread awareness and understanding. Most of all, thank you to my wonderful husband for all your knowledge, editing, input, and support. I could not imagine being on this journey without you by my side.

DISCLAIMER

I am not a doctor or medical professional. The information provided in this book is for educational or informational purposes only. I am not providing healthcare services, or attempting to diagnose, treat, or cure any physical, mental, or emotional issue, disease, or condition. Although I strive to provide accurate information, the information presented throughout this book is not intended to be a substitute for medical advice, diagnosis, or treatment by your own medical provider. Always seek the advice of a medical professional regarding any questions or concerns about your health.

TABLE OF CONTENTS

DAY 1:
My Story

I used to avoid talking about my pain. I don't like to complain, and I know that everyone has challenges in life. So I suffered in silence for over a decade. As I slowly began to open up, people came out of the shadows. I realized that I wasn't alone in feeling alone and that by sharing my story, I gained new opportunities to offer support and encouragement to others.

I now firmly believe that if I want people to understand something, then it's my job to teach them (with patience and kindness). I can't expect others to do what I won't. Of course, not everyone is willing to listen; but if I don't at least try, then I'm not even giving them the opportunity. For that reason, I've been more open about my pain. I try to represent my life truthfully, instead of constantly putting on the picture-perfect, social media mask.

Pain is nothing new for me. As a former gymnast, it's instinctive for me to push my body to its limits and hide any pain. After all, I couldn't grimace and groan during my routines, and I definitely didn't want to sit on the sidelines. When I was diagnosed with arthritis at age 18, it just seemed like par for the course. It was the price I had to pay for asking my joints to do unnatural things for so many years. Then after I got married, I had two extremely difficult pregnancies and learned that I have an estrogen intolerance—something I had never heard of before. I was incredibly sick throughout the entire pregnancies, lost 25 pounds, and had an at-home IV. However, when there's an end in sight (9 months) and a positive goal (baby), it's easier to find the motivation to make it through each day.

Then about a year after my first child was born, migraines became a part of my life, and the real struggle began. A migraine is more than just a bad headache. Besides the severe head throbbing, it's often accompanied by nausea, vomiting, extreme sensitivity to light and sound, mental confusion, and so much more. Migraine attacks can last for days and completely debilitate the sufferer. I gave up caffeine (including chocolate), which seemed to help for a little while. But after my migraines increased again, I started searching desperately for an answer. I eliminated dairy and gluten from my diet and began the discouraging process of being passed from doctor to doctor.

I was diagnosed with a vestibular imbalance. Our balance comes from a combination of vestibular input, sensory awareness, and vision. As long as any two of these are working, you should be fairly balanced. Since my vestibular input is compromised, my balance is dependent on both my sensory awareness and sight. So, if I'm standing, I fall over when I close my eyes. I went through almost a year of physical therapy, but it never improved and soon became the scapegoat for all of my symptoms.

At this point, pain changed from an unwelcome visitor to a permanent resident. Even on my migraine-free days, I still had a persistent headache. Dizziness, blurred vision, fatigue, and light sensitivity decided to join the party as well. More than 15 years after my migraines first started, I was spending about five days a week in bed, and prescription medication was required for me to complete simple daily activities. Finally, after trying more than 18 prescriptions and seeing 10 different doctors, I had a diagnosis. A fairly large cyst had been growing in the middle of my brain. Because of the cyst's location, only a handful of neurosurgeons in the United States were capable of and willing to remove it.

After five months and being in communication with four different neurosurgeons across the country, the day arrived. It sounds strange to say, but even though I was heading into an incredibly invasive and risky surgery, I wasn't nervous at all. I knew that everything up to that point had led me there and that things just couldn't keep going the way they were. I wasn't living; I was simply existing.

I'm not going to lie: recovery wasn't easy or quick. However, the moment that I woke up from surgery, my constant headache was gone. I no longer felt and heard my pulse in my head. I went from migraines five days a week to six or seven days a month. My blurred vision and dizzy spells rarely show their unwelcome face anymore. It's been six years now and even though I still have limitations and am always in some level of pain, I'm thankful for how far I've come. Looking at computer and phone screens for extended periods of time increases my migraines so, ironically, writing a book about pain causes me more pain.

Three years after my brain surgery, I started to have gastrointestinal issues and found myself on an entirely new pain journey. After several tests, my gastroenterologist suggested that it was probably IBS (irritable bowel syndrome). But nothing really helped and my health continued to decline. Upon waking each day, my entire midsection felt bruised but appeared normal. By the time I went to bed at night, I looked to be about six months pregnant. It felt like all my organs were tied in a knot and wrapped in barbed wire. It was exhausting, and I couldn't make it through a day without a nap. I often skipped meals because of the pain. It became difficult to breathe sometimes. My chest was tight and my joints ached. I hated leaving the house, not only because of the pain, but because my self-esteem had plummeted. I liked being active and fit. Even through all my previous struggles, I'd been able to maintain my body shape. However, there was nothing I could do about this belly bloat. Pants that fit in the morning would be painfully tight by the afternoon, and it became more difficult to hide the bulge. It was mentally, emotionally, and physically draining.

After seeing four different doctors and having multiple tests over a couple of years, a nurse practitioner suggested that I look into endometriosis. I had heard of that but didn't really know much about it. Endometriosis is a disease where tissue similar to the uterine lining grows outside the womb. The longer that it goes undiagnosed, the more damage it can do. It can spread to the bowel, bladder, intestines, joints, diaphragm, and rarely even to the heart and lungs. It spiderwebs out and can fuse organs together. Lesions often grow deep into the tissue. This disease literally mutilates you on the inside. It's estimated that it affects 10 percent of women, although it's impossible to know the exact number because the only way to definitively diagnose it is with surgery. It rarely shows up on scans, and takes an average of seven to nine years and eight different doctors to get a diagnosis. Most women are dismissed as neurotic, told that their symptoms are normal, or misdiagnosed with something else. Because of my past, I've learned to trust my instincts and fight for an answer. I already knew what it was like to be dismissed as overexaggerating by doctor after doctor. But I'm not a hypochondriac, and I actually have a very high pain tolerance.

So I found a specialist and prepared for another surgery. I was more nervous about this one. As strange as it sounds, I was terrified that he wouldn't find anything wrong and I'd be back to square one. I think only people living with unanswered chronic pain can truly understand that. As it turns out, I did have significant endometriosis that had spread to other organs. While excision (cutting out the bad tissue and lesions) is the best treatment course, if any endometrial cells are missed, they often continue to spread. After my excision, many of my symptoms went away for a few months, but then they started to return. Seven months later, I ended up having a hysterectomy. They found more endometriosis, adenomyosis, and some growths. I'm still recovering from that surgery and hoping that I'll finally find some relief.

That leads us to this book. I now feel it's important for me to share my health challenges because it's still considered taboo by many. It's personal. We don't want to seem needy and weak or we've been wounded too many times by those who don't believe us. As a result, there are people all around us who are silently suffering. And maybe if we talked more openly, I would've found answers sooner. If my being vulnerable helps even one person, then it's totally worth it. Trust your instincts when something is wrong. It's not normal to live in pain. My hope is that this book shows people that they aren't alone and gives them a quick and easy-to-read resource to help others understand what it's like to live with chronic pain.

DAY 2:
What Is Chronic Pain?

There are many synonyms for *pain* in the English language: suffering, agony, affliction, torture, torment, discomfort, soreness, ache, hurt, or misery. And there are even more adjectives to describe it: aching, stinging, burning, stabbing, cramping, pressure, splitting, gnawing, sharp, shooting, tender, throbbing, and so on. Yet somehow all these words often seem inadequate.

Pain is a warning that something is wrong. Whether it is caused by a virus, touching something hot, a broken bone, or cancer, pain's role is to protect us. It is vital for survival because it motivates us to take action—to withdraw, flee, rest, change our habits, or seek medical treatment. Without pain, the world becomes a dreadfully dangerous place.

Congenital insensitivity to pain, also known as *congenital analgesia*, is hereditary and makes a person incapable of sensing pain or temperature. While this rare disease might seem like a blessing in disguise, it can lead to a shorter life expectancy. Imagine a child repeatedly getting burned, biting off the tip of their tongue, or breaking bones without even noticing. It is common for people with this condition to not live past childhood due to ignored injuries, infections, or illnesses.

Chronic pain can be difficult to define. It is complex and varies from person to person. Pain is usually a symptom of an injury or illness. If you stub your toe or pull a muscle, you feel discomfort that corresponds with that specific injury. This is *acute pain*, and it goes away once the underlying cause is healed.

On the other hand, sometimes pain extends beyond the expected healing time. Maybe it never went away or it continually returns. Many experts describe *chronic pain* as pain that is present every day for more than 3 months or is present on more than 50 percent of days for 6 months. It is long term and far more frustrating than acute pain—coping with any affliction for an extended period of time is challenging. Chronic pain can come in many forms, from a dull nuisance to searing agony, and is divided into four broad categories:

> **1.** *Nociceptive*—This is the most common and is caused by harm to the body. When your skin, muscles, bones, ligaments, or other tissues get damaged, nociceptors (sensory receptors) notify your brain about the injury. After your brain receives the signal, it interprets the information and perceives that there is pain. When the cause of pain gets stronger, the nociceptors shoot off signals more rapidly and intensely, but weaker messages are given less priority. This prevents your brain from overreacting to a minor scrape. Normally these receptors only activate when there is an illness or injury

and then stop once the area has healed.
However, sometimes the nociceptors send
signals even after the injury is gone, causing chronic pain. Nociceptive pain has
two sub categories: somatic and visceral.

Somatic pain comes from external factors,
such as a laceration or broken bone. It
is typically caused by force, temperature,
or swelling and is often localized to a
particular area. Muscle soreness after
exercising is not chronic pain; but if
the post-workout ache continues longer
than the expected healing time, then it
is chronic somatic muscle pain. Examples of somatic pain include arthritis,
osteoporosis, tendonitis, bruises, and a
sprained ankle.

Visceral pain is triggered by internal organs,
such as pelvic pain due to a bladder infection or abdominal pain caused by IBS
(irritable bowel syndrome). The trouble
with visceral pain is that the brain cannot
always pinpoint the problem area. Our
internal organs do not have as many nociceptors as the skin, which makes it difficult for our brains to figure out exactly
where the pain originated. For example,
pain in the lower back could be a sign
that something is wrong with the kidneys.

This is called referred pain. Examples of visceral pain include endometriosis, heart attack, and appendicitis.

2. *Neuropathic*—This is caused by nerves not functioning normally, due to irritation, damage, or malfunction. Our bodies contain a network of nerves that weave in and out of the spinal column and then branch out to other parts of the body in order to transmit pain indicators to our brains. If these nerves get damaged, they will send out faulty signals. This can happen when a nerve gets crushed during an injury. If the nerve damage remains after the wound has healed, the result is neuropathic chronic pain. Neuropathic pain can also be the result of dysfunctional nerves that misfire. This may appear to come out of nowhere, rather than from a specific injury. It can also cause you to feel discomfort in response to things that are usually not painful, such as cold air or clothing against your skin. Examples of neuropathic pain include Bell's palsy, multiple sclerosis, diabetic neuropathy, and sciatica.

3. *Psychogenic*—This is the term used for pain caused by a psychological disorder, such as depression or anxiety. There is some disagreement among experts about whether or not chronic pain can have a purely mental or emotional origin. However, many do agree that stress or emotional distress can cause physical complications, such as fatigue, muscle aches, headaches, or nausea. People with psychogenic pain are often stigmatized by those who believe the pain is not real; this may include both medical professionals and the general public. Because it does not seem to have a physical origin, psychogenic pain is more difficult to diagnose and treat than nociceptive or neuropathic pain.

4. *Idiopathic*—This is pain that exists when there is no known physical or psychological cause. It may be idiopathic from the start or become that way over time, such as pain that lingers long after an injury has healed and no tissue or nerve damage can be found. While the cause may not be detectable with current medical knowledge, the pain is still very real. This is extremely frustrating for both doctors and sufferers and can lead to never-ending tests and continually changing treatments. Without an apparent source, it is difficult to diagnose and treat this type of pain. Examples of idiopathic pain include TMJ or TMD (temporomandibular joint disorders), IBS, "ice-pick" headaches, and fibromyalgia.

No matter the type of pain, you likely just want it to stop hurting. With such different categories, it is important to accurately describe your pain in order to give your doctor the best chance of properly diagnosing and treating the problem.

CHRONIC PAIN CATEGORIES

NOCICEPTIVE
· Caused by harm to the body

NEUROPATHIC
· Caused by nerves not functioning normally

PSYCHOGENIC
· Caused by psychological disorder

IDIOPATHIC
· No known physical or psychological cause

DAY 3:
Cost

Chronic pain is expensive. It is incorrect to think of it as just long-lasting acute pain. Once it becomes chronic, it takes on a life of its own and is often difficult to stop. This can lead to surgeries, injections, therapies, supplements, and numerous different medications. Many patients are willing to try almost anything for some relief, but it is usually challenging to find something that is truly effective. At best, these treatments tend to provide a temporary respite. I have often said that I would wear a live chicken on my head if it would cure my migraines.

Chronic, unrelieved pain affects millions of Americans and is growing in prevalence (Day 15). It is costly both financially and in the toll that it takes on people's lives. It is economically burdensome on not only the affected individuals, but their families and friends, their employers, and the nation as a whole. A National Academy of Sciences 2010 study found that in the United States, the yearly economic cost of chronic pain is $635 billion—and it has likely increased since then. This estimate includes the cost of health care ($300 billion) and the cost of missed work ($335 billion).[1] That is higher than the annual costs for cancer, heart disease, and diabetes. Medicare bears one-fourth of the U.S. medical expenses for chronic pain. In 2008, chronic pain cost federal and state programs $99 billion, and this did not include lost tax revenues due to missed work and lower wages. This study also acknowledged that the estimates are likely conservative because the figures do not account for certain segments of the population.

There are a number of factors that go into the high cost of chronic pain. Many patients receive inadequate pain prevention, diagnoses, and treatment. This is in part because of unrealistic patient expectations, the need for individualized care, and a lack of sufficient assessment and treatment methods (Day 13). This increases the number of visits, doctors, and medications that sufferers are willing to try. As a result, many people who suffer from chronic pain start looking for alternatives when they feel that conventional medicine has failed them.

While not included in the costs discussed above, there is no shortage of nonpharmacological options out there. From compression clothing and patches to acupuncture and massage to yoga and electrical nerve stimulation (like TENS units) to supplements and topical rubs. Though some people can find relief in these treatments, most are not covered by insurance and the out-of-pocket cost can be very expensive. For example, massage or acupuncture can be well over $100 per visit. Since these kinds of therapies usually involve repeat visits, they often end up costing patients thousands of dollars in order to achieve any long-term benefit. Purchasing braces, Kinesiology Therapeutic (KT) Tape, oils, or supplements can also add up quickly. And since the human body is so complex, treatments that work for one person can be ineffective or even harmful for someone else.

According to a 2012 survey, Americans spent $30.2 billion out of pocket on complementary health approaches.[2] Yet since many people with chronic pain struggle with missed work or lower wages, they are often unable to afford these alternative treatments—especially when combined with the cost of their regular medications or therapies that do offer a small measure of relief. So every alternative option purchased, even for a trial period, requires a financial investment and is a gamble. If the product or therapy is not helpful at all, then the sufferer has wasted even more money. It can be a difficult choice—a possible respite from the suffering versus the potential for yet another expensive failure. The journey to find the best combination of treatments is often long and full of uncertainty.

HEALTH CARE
~ $300 billion

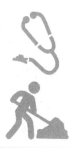

LOST PRODUCTIVITY
~ $335 billion

ANNUAL U.S. COST
OF CHRONIC PAIN
~ $635 billion

DAY 4:
Invisible Illnesses

What is a chronic illness? According to the US National Center for Health Statistics, a chronic illness is a disease that lasts for three months or longer. Usually, vaccines cannot prevent them and medications cannot cure them, nor do they just disappear. The most prominent are cardiovascular diseases, cancer, chronic obstructive pulmonary disease (COPD), and type 2 diabetes. According to the World Health Organization (WHO), chronic diseases are the leading cause of death and disability worldwide.[3] Their 2002 report indicated that chronic illness accounts for nearly 60 percent of all global deaths.

So what is an invisible illness then? This is an umbrella term for any medical condition that is not visible to others—including fibromyalgia, headache disorders, Lyme disease, traumatic brain injuries, as well as mental illnesses. Often there are no signs that can be seen with scans or blood tests, but the symptoms of these invisible illnesses do exist.

Having an illness that is invisible often leads to judgment and criticism, especially if the individual is young (Day 17). Because they may look healthy on the outside, others tend to be skeptical (Day 24). Sufferers often get accused of being lazy or rude, faking it, or having it all be in their heads (Day 19). They frequently have to justify resting, staying home, taking medications, continually fidgeting or changing positions to get comfortable, or using handicap parking. From the outside looking in, this can be difficult to understand. And from the inside looking out, it is often difficult to explain.

To complicate things even more, invisible illness symptoms often ebb and flow—some hours, days, or even months go pretty well and other times it becomes almost impossible to work, socialize, or function. For healthy people, this can be confusing. Sometimes they *prescribe* things like, "Just think positively…Take a nap…Go out and have some fun…Drink more water…" While the motives may be pure, comments like these are dismissive. They minimize the individual's diagnosis and make them feel alone (Day 18).

On top of already dealing with their condition, many patients have the additional burden of needing to constantly advocate for themselves and explain their illness to others (Day 6). This not only includes friends and family, but sometimes medical professionals as well (Day 13).

When an illness or injury is visible, people tend to be more understanding of the limitations. They can see and comprehend a neck brace, wheelchair, or oxygen tank. Imagine someone entering an elevator in a wheelchair. Most people will be helpful, patient, and kind—little to no irritation or disapproving looks. Now picture someone else sluggishly exiting that same elevator on foot. Do you think this person will receive the same accommodations from the crowd? The inflamed joints causing agonizing pain with every step are not visible. Thanks to vertigo, no one else can see the walls spinning. They cannot even see the last bit of energy being used up for this seemingly simple task. When people cannot see your impairment or condition, they assume that you should have no difficulty performing everyday tasks. This, of course, is far from the truth.

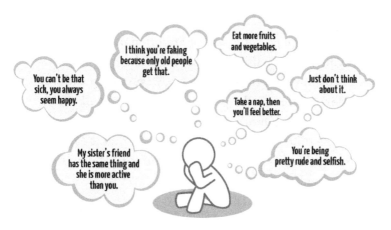

DAY 5:
Thoughts, Emotions, and Behavior

Chronic pain involves physical, mental, and emotional factors. After the nerves send out the physical pain signals (Day 2), the brain assesses them along with the surrounding events. These thoughts then influence how the pain is perceived. For example, general body aches after a vigorous workout are seen as good pain. However, similar aches are understood as bad when they are the result of a medical condition, such as fibromyalgia.

Even though *pain* and *suffering* are often used as synonyms, it is our thoughts that make the difference. A broken bone, for example, may cause pain without suffering because the person knows that it will heal and is nothing more than a temporary inconvenience. On the other hand, similar bone pain that is caused by a tumor may result in increased suffering due to the meaning behind it.

Our emotions follow our thoughts. When we believe the pain is not dangerous or fatal, then our emotional response is usually minimal. However, if we think the pain is a serious threat, like cancer, then we may respond with fear, stress, anger, anxiety, or depression (Day 20). In addition, when the pain steals our entire focus, it limits our outside interests and distractions. This can lead to feelings of hopelessness, resentment, or loneliness (Day 18). Our pain is intimately linked to our emotions, and our emotions influence our behaviors.

Some pain behaviors are as simple as talking about it, grimacing, or moving slowly—and these can be based on the environment. For example, you may try to hide your symptoms more at work than you do at home. Then there are other behaviors that have more serious consequences, such as breaking apart relationships or taking the enjoyment out of life. These include things like withdrawing from social situations, becoming irritable or unresponsive, avoiding activities that you used to enjoy, having suicidal thoughts, exaggerating grunting and groaning, or making unnecessary demands on family, friends, or coworkers.

When chronic illness makes it difficult to live a full and productive life, the person is often left feeling isolated and alone (Day 18). This is frequently compounded if the sufferer has little to no support system (Day 29). In some situations, it can be helpful to seek a mental health professional who is experienced in treating patients with chronic conditions. Many therapists even offer virtual sessions, which can make it easier for those who struggle to leave their homes. Mental health plays an important role in physical health.

Cognitive behavioral therapy (CBT) can help some people develop skills to change the negative thoughts and behaviors in order to cope better, even when the actual level of pain stays the same. Its aim is to help the patient modify the way they view their pain. While they may not be able to control the pain itself, they can take control of how they deal with it.

PHYSICAL
Pain, Fatigue

THOUGHTS
I'm all alone. This
will never end

BEHAVIOR
Isolation, Missed
Work, Lashing Out

EMOTIONS
Fear, Anger, Anxiety,
Depression

DAY 6:
Lack of Understanding

With the exception of patients who have congenital analgesia (Day 2), everyone experiences some degree of pain at some point. This can make it difficult for many people to understand how chronic pain is different than the familiar acute pain which they have felt. A healthy person might assume that it is like having a cold or a sore muscle that just hangs around, but they struggle to fully comprehend the ups and downs. It is more like being trapped on a never-ending rollercoaster for the rest of your life. There are moments when it slows down and you try to catch your breath, but you know that the big drop and dark tunnel are right around the corner. And no matter how sick or tired you become, you can never get off.

A strange thing happens when you become hurt or sick with something that will not go away anytime soon. Communicating exactly how you feel becomes an almost impossible task. How do you explain that your body, and even your mind, regularly betray you? That you feel alone (Day 18), guilty (Day 10), useless, and misunderstood—sometimes while simultaneously smiling, laughing, and finding enjoyment? That there is not any visible evidence proving you are sick (Day 4)? When there is no way to adequately explain the burden that you carry, loneliness and depression (Day 20) sneak up on you.

People also frequently fail to understand what *chronic* really means. It is not uncommon for sufferers to hear things like, "I hope you get better soon." While this is well-intentioned, it can be difficult to know how to respond. In reality, there will probably be days when you *feel* a little better (Day 27), but you are unlikely to ever actually *get* better. The severity of the symptoms can ebb and flow, but once pain becomes chronic, it is often for life.

When pain is attributed to a well-known and culturally accepted disease, like cancer, it is usually believed, treated with real concern, and considered valid. However, when the underlying issue is lesser known or not well-defined, like chronic fatigue syndrome, it is not uncommon for patients to be ignored by not only friends and family but also health care professionals (Day 13). Reactions can range from care and compassion to complete dismissal and accusations against the sufferer. The more a disease is misunderstood, the less believed the symptoms become. When something cannot be seen or measured objectively (Day 4), it is more likely to be disregarded, avoided, or attributed to overreaction, emotional instability, or worse. The irony is that this pain and suffering are no less than that of patients with well-known ailments—yet the cultural perception is dramatically different.

It is not uncommon for even friends or family to become nervous when they ask how you are doing. Words like *pain*, *despair*, or *suffering* can make many people uncomfortable. Yet these are part of everyday life for chronic pain patients. Not ever being able to voice one's true thoughts has psychological consequences and fuels the misunderstanding about both the condition and the person who lives with it.

Sometimes when people do open up about their pain challenges, they are confronted with sentiments such as, "It's not really that bad. It could always be worse." Those are often followed up with a compare-and-contrast story about someone else. This makes the person regret ever mentioning it and feel like they are just complaining. Everyone wants to be heard and understood, especially when the road they are on is rocky with no end in sight. Yet many people do not think of chronic illness as being serious; they see it more as a minor irritant that can be resolved simply by going to the doctor or taking medication. Open communication helps break the stigmas (Day 7) and eliminates needless misunderstandings.

LIVING WITH CHRONIC PAIN

(physical or mental) can feel like being trapped in a hole by yourself.

DOCTORS: That's normal.
FAMILY & FRIENDS: What hole? You seem fine.
BOSS: Take a sick day. That will help.
GOVERNMENT: Sorry, there's a waiting list for ladders.
WHAT I NEED: I see you and am coming down there. I won't let you try to climb out by yourself.

DAY 7:
Breaking the Stigmas

Misconceptions about chronic illness increase the weight of the burden and often cause people to hide their ailment. While it is vital to be able to explain your condition, the fear of being misunderstood (Day 6) and not believed scares many people into silence. Yet without having open conversations, the stigmas will never change.

The Oxford Dictionary gives a definition of *stigma* as "a mark of disgrace associated with a particular circumstance, quality, or person." And it can be cruel. It labels people as outside the norm—different and tainted. It happens quickly and is often done unconsciously. Ironically, it is not the health condition itself that stigmatizes people; it is other people.

"He never hangs out anymore." In addition to regular pain and exhaustion, some ailments are aggravated by certain environments, like loud restaurants or bright lights. These things can lead to the assumption that the person is rude, unapproachable, or reclusive. As a result, some people will withdraw from social events and isolate themselves even further.

"She's not that sick." It is easy to forget that pain can sometimes be managed enough to function socially. This does not mean that they are faking it. In fact, it is not uncommon for many sufferers to fake being well. Just because a person looks normal does not mean that they feel normal or are able to do normal things (Day 24).

"Don't look at him. He has a disability." There are conditions that society views as untouchable—the "Shh, don't ask" issues. People avert their eyes and teach their kids not to engage in conversation because they fear the unknown. This makes the sufferer feel even more alone and ostracized.

"Why won't she tell me what's wrong?" Many conditions have embarrassing or taboo symptoms—like severe constipation or diarrhea, excessive sweating, painful bloating, or dangerously heavy menstrual bleeding. As a result, many people suffer in silence.

"That's the guy with the really weird disease." Living with a chronic illness can mean whispers and judgment from others. People watch closely and sometimes point. Others may be afraid that it is contagious. Employers can be leery of hiring someone so sick. All this can cause feelings of shame (Day 10) and anxiety.

"She can't have that. She's too young." Some people view youth and chronic pain as opposites (Day 17). After all, health problems are typically short term and curable for young people. But the pain and suffering are not any less real just because someone is under a certain age.

"He's so lazy." Many chronic ailments are more than debilitating—they are also exhausting (Days 8 and 12). This often goes beyond the symptoms themselves; the aftereffects can leave the sufferer drained for days (Day 27). However, instead of taking the time to rest, many will struggle internally in order to pretend that everything is fine. This is often out of fear that others will not believe that there is anything wrong.

"We always have to go to her house. She never comes to ours." Leaving the house can be difficult and exhausting for those with chronic illnesses. Every individual task requires effort and drains the person's energy supply—showering, getting dressed, doing hair and makeup, driving, getting gas, socializing, etc. And then if they do run out of energy, getting back home can seem like an impossible mission (Day 8).

"He never eats with us anymore." Food is an integral part of social gatherings. However, many chronic conditions have their own recommended diet. Certain foods exacerbate pain and can trigger flare-ups. People living with chronic pain often have unusual eating habits or skip meals altogether, which may seem strange or unhealthy to others.

While stigmas like these can be painful and exhausting, remaining silent does not make them any less so. No one should be shamed when their pain causes them to move a little slower. Nobody should be made to feel guilty when their illness causes them to miss social events. No one should be embarrassed when they need the handicap seat, parking, or other services. And nobody should be afraid to talk about their chronic pain or illness.

As human beings, it can be difficult to understand things that are outside our sphere of experience. We can imagine how we might feel or act, but we cannot truly know. So if we have any hope of breaking the stigmas and spreading awareness, we need to be able to communicate openly when the opportunities present themselves. It is also crucial to remember that people are more than their pain, illness, or disability.

BREAK
THE STIGMA

Useless PAIN
Exhaustion Medications
Poor Sleep Disappointment
Frustration Inflammation
Helplessness Guilt Lack of Understanding
Alone   Strained Relationships Anxiety
Negative Self-Image Uncomfortable
Brain Fog Suffering Decreased Activity
Silence   Costs Missed Work
Achy   Disabilities
Irritability

DAY 8:
Spoon Theory

Being able to explain chronic pain and illness is essential to eliminating misunderstandings (Days 6 and 7), but that is easier said than done. And some days are better than others, with varying levels of pain and energy. Have you ever heard someone say that they were out of spoons for the day or that they did not have enough spoons left to complete something? If you do not live with a chronic illness, that terminology probably sounds strange to you.

Spoon theory is a tool for helping people understand how someone with a chronic condition gets worn down. It has become a popular concept and was created by Christine Miserandino in 2003.[4] She was out to dinner with a friend and was asked to explain what living with her illness is like. Christine, who has lupus, grabbed 12 spoons and handed them to her friend. Imagining that the spoons represented her limited pool of energy, she explained that every task she performs requires a spoon. Get out of bed—remove a spoon. Put on clothes—remove another spoon. Cook a meal—there goes more. Every activity has a price.

Once there were only six spoons left and her friend had not even gone to work yet, there was a glimpse of understanding. Christine then explained that her friend needed to choose the rest of her day carefully. Once the spoons are gone, so is the energy. Sometimes you can borrow from the next day's supply, but that means you will start tomorrow with a deficit. It is also important to note that this comes with a high interest rate. If you borrow one to get through the rest of today, it may actually cost you two or three of tomorrow's spoons. After things like vacations or special occasions, you may be out of spoons for days. Because this penalty is nonnegotiable, budgeting your spoons is crucial.

All of this forced Christine's friend to start thinking differently about the rest of her make-believe day. With only one spoon left, she just did not have enough remaining energy to do everything she wanted. Sometimes you have to ration your spoons in order to complete more draining tasks, which means that other areas of your life will suffer. But you simply cannot go over your limit of spoons.

Strategic spoon management—or pacing (Day 27)—is important because the only way you can refill them is by resting. And some days you may wake up with fewer than normal or even a couple of extra ones. It is often unpredictable. Spoonie (what chronically ill people sometimes refer to themselves as) rest is not laziness. On the other hand, you need to subtract some spoons if you did not sleep well, forgot to take your medication, or got sick. You always have to be aware of your energy balance and figure out what your priorities are.

Because there is no medical jargon and it is not specific to one chronic illness, this analogy has become a nice and easy tool for anyone to use. It is also an effective visual. People can better understand something that is outside their sphere of experience when they can visualize it. That is why spoon theory works so well.

However, if spoon theory does not really make much sense to you, try imagining your energy like a bank account. While healthy people have substantial and stable accounts, chronic pain patients carry low balances because they live paycheck to paycheck (i.e., rest to rest). You can save your money (energy) or spend it. But if you use more than what is in your account, you will find yourself in debt. For someone with a chronic illness, each morning might reveal a different balance. Occasionally you wake up to find an unexpected bonus while other mornings you discover that you are broke—even though you did not spend it all the day before. It is almost like a thief hacked your account overnight. No matter how hard you try not to spend it all, it disappears so quickly and you can never really get ahead.

Both of these analogies are simplistic, imperfect, and do not even begin to address other major chronic ailment symptoms, but they can help explain what it is like to live with low energy storage. Healthy people are able to start their day with innumerable possibilities. They have enough energy to do pretty much anything they want. They are able to go about their busy schedules with little to no pain or discomfort. They can complete normal daily tasks without having to worry about severe exhaustion.

We live in such a fast-paced world and there is always so much to do. For chronic illness sufferers, one of the hardest lessons to learn is to slow down because you cannot do everything. It is easy to feel guilty (Day 10), lazy, or left out. It is difficult to leave projects unfinished and to stay home when everyone else is out having fun. But once your body informs you that you are done, you need to rest and stop comparing yourself to others. When you rest because your body is weak, you are not wasting time doing nothing. You are doing exactly what you need to do. You are recovering.

SPOON THEORY

Imagine starting each day with only 12–15 spoons.
How would you spend them?

GET OUT OF BED	SHOWER	MAKE AND EAT A MEAL	GO TO WORK OR SCHOOL
GET DRESSED	DO HAIR AND MAKEUP	WALK THE DOG	HOUSEWORK
BRUSH TEETH	MAKE PLANS	DRIVE	SHOPPING
WATCH TV	READ OR STUDY	SOCIALIZE	EXERCISE

DAY 9:
The Pain Scale

Pain is personal. Nobody else can perceive your pain through their senses. Unlike heart murmurs, it cannot be heard. It cannot be seen with X-rays. While lumps can be felt with touch, pain cannot. It also has no taste or smell. Currently, there is no clinical test for pain. It is a subjective experience. What feels excruciating to one person may feel mild to someone else. Symptoms can vary in duration and intensity, and they are highly individualized. This can make it difficult to find the appropriate treatment for each distinct patient.

Doctors use standard metrics to assess your vital signs. They do not just ask you if you have a fever or high blood pressure; they use a thermometer and a cuff to run their own tests. Your body temperature, blood pressure, pulse, and oxygen level are objective numbers. They give insights about your current level of wellness. However, pain is measured and evaluated by the patients themselves, based on their own metrics. This is completely subjective. Because we all experience pain differently, there is no real standard.

Most of us are familiar with this. We find ourselves at a clinic or hospital and the doctor asks, "On a scale of zero to ten, what is your level of pain? Zero being no pain and ten being the worst that you have ever experienced." On the surface, this seems like an easy enough question to answer, but is it really?

The doctor will likely use your response to determine whether or not your complaint is urgent. So, your mind races. *Will they even care if it has only been a solid three or four for months, but is still affecting my daily life? What if my eight sounds like I am lying in order to get drugs? Will the difference between a four and a six change the treatment I receive?* You are being asked to define your entire pain experience with a single number. And healthcare providers are only human. Their biases will inevitably influence how they view this one answer. You might be believed and taken seriously, treated as if you are overreacting and exaggerating, or viewed as a drug addict attempting to get narcotics (Day 25).

Beyond that, remember that pain is relative. Two people with the same broken leg might give completely different ratings, even though neither can stand or move the limb on its own. The number scale is also particularly difficult for many men because, while talking to a doctor or nurse, they tend to downplay how much things hurt. In addition, this scale cannot account for people who are always in some level of pain. Pain operates differently for people with chronic issues. What was once an eight or nine, becomes a three or four after living with it for a while. On good days, some people can actually forget about the pain, even though it is still there. The longer that someone is in constant pain, the better they become at ignoring it. They get used to it and learn to tune out the lower levels. At some point, they need to keep on living despite it because they cannot writhe around on the floor or stay in bed every day, no matter how much they want to. They often learn how to go about life with a smile—and most people are none the wiser. This can be an additional problem when sitting with a doctor because the nonverbal cues that they normally look for are absent. So what does the pain scale even mean for someone who experiences chronic pain? What is the baseline? Is exhaustion considered painful (Days 8 and 12)? It is worth noting that the pain scale can be helpful for therapists or other health professionals who monitor the patient on a regular basis. Frequently comparing the individual's pain levels over a period of time is one of the easiest ways to determine how much progress, if any, is being made.

Chronic pain is complex. With no set standard, it can be difficult to describe because words often seem inadequate. And yet accurately describing it is essential for doctors to find the cause and the right treatment. Instead of focusing on a number, explain the following to your doctor: what it is like living with it, what it prevents you from doing, what you have tried that made it better or worse, how long you have had it, and how often it occurs. These answers not only help with a diagnosis and treatment plan but also in determining support and service options.

It can be helpful to write those details down before your appointment. Recording your daily symptoms can help as well—this will show your doctor when your pain waxes and wanes. The pain scale only gives a point-in-time reading, whereas tracking your symptoms over days or weeks gives a more complete picture. And remember that your goal may not be to get to zero; it might just be small wins that allow you to experience life again.

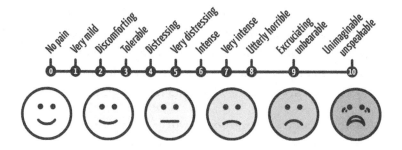

DAY 10:
Guilt and Shame

In addition to the physical symptoms, it is common for chronic conditions to cause feelings of guilt and shame. This may sound strange or confusing to those who do not suffer from a chronic illness. After all, why would anyone feel guilty for being ill? Yet it seems nearly unavoidable to experience chronic pain that is not accompanied by some level of guilt.

When it comes to awareness, words like *fighter*, *warrior*, *thriver*, or *conqueror* become part of the conversation. But in the reality of daily life, carrying this heavy burden can make it difficult to feel like a champion. In fact, you often feel frustrated, exhausted (Day 12), forgetful (Day 14), and completely defeated. Life's responsibilities remain the same, but you have limits that you may not have had before. Overcoming the guilt is difficult when it feels like you are always letting everyone, including yourself, down. And for some people, this can actually be worse than the illness itself and can include:

> - Physical Guilt – *I am a burden*. Everyone would like to be fast, energetic, strong, and capable. However, chronic pain can be debilitating and often makes you less able. Because of this, it asks a great deal from caretakers, family, and friends, which can be draining for them as well.

- Household Guilt – *I do not contribute enough*. This may seem the same as physical guilt, but it deserves its own category. Daily household chores are essential for a home to run smoothly. And being incapable of doing these tasks regularly, or at all, affects everyone in the house.

- Social Guilt – *I am constantly letting down the people I love*. Chronic illnesses can be unpredictable, and you never know how you will feel from day to day (Day 23). This leads to canceled plans and missed social activities.

- Financial Guilt – *My illness is too expensive for my family*. The cost of chronic pain can be massive (Day 3), and it is often difficult for the sufferer to contribute to the household income.

- Work Guilt – *I have to call in sick again*. Chronic illnesses can make you feel bad for not only disappointing your friends and family but also your boss and co-workers.

- Food Guilt – *I make everything more difficult*. Many people bond over food, but strict dietary restrictions play a big role in managing chronic pain. Food and restaurant options are often quite limited. Guilt creeps in when you feel like you are always controlling where to eat or what to serve.

- Medication Guilt – *I should be able to manage my pain better. Am I making myself worse by taking so many medications? Are they even really working?* Unrealistic expectations can cause patients to doubt their treatments. Between preventative medications to reduce the frequency and abortive medications to lessen the symptoms once they start, it is easy to question everything when your chronic illness never goes away—even though logically you know that it never will.

- Undiagnosis Guilt – *What is wrong with me? Maybe I am crazy.* This can be one of the most difficult. When you do not have a diagnosis, you feel lost. With no answer, there is no course of action and it becomes increasingly difficult to stay optimistic. Living in the unknown can make you wonder if you are actually imagining it all (Day 19).

- Partner Guilt – *My spouse does not deserve this.* Chronic illness affects every relationship. However, a partnership is often expected to be equal, so it can be difficult when one person cannot regularly fulfill their role. When this happens, the relationship can feel one sided, even when the other person is understanding and does not complain.

- Parenting Guilt – *My kids deserve better than me.* It hurts whenever any parent misses big and small moments in the lives of their kids. But there is an added layer of guilt when the only reason for it is your chronic illness. Then there is the guilt of overburdening your children with extra responsibilities and worries.

Guilt is a feeling of responsibility or remorse. Whether real or imagined, these feelings can lead to other negative consequences—such as anxiety, depression (Day 20), isolation, increased pain, a weakened immune system, and shame.

Shame is a painful feeling of humiliation or distress caused by the belief that one's behavior or experiences are wrong, foolish, or dishonorable. This a useful emotion when it protects us from violating our values. It acts as a brake or a moral compass. It teaches us to use restraint or caution when we fall short, and it exposes our weak spots. The good news is that we can only feel shame if we have a conscience that is working properly.

However, when shame is allowed to take root and grow, it makes you feel worthless and inadequate. Feeling guilty for the things that you are unable to do can trigger feelings of shame over who you are. This can prevent you from experiencing future interests, excitement, or joy. Once this happens, your pain is no longer just about your malfunctioning body, it is about your character or your identity as a person. It is somehow your fault for getting and staying sick. At best, you feel incompetent or useless. At worst, you feel like there is no point to your existence—like the world would be better without you in it.

For that reason, learning to identify and manage guilt is essential for anyone living with chronic pain. The reality is that you may not ever fully overcome these feelings, but you can get through them. You have to accept that it is not your fault when your body betrays you. You are not responsible for things that are out of your control. It is possible to acknowledge your guilt, let it go, and then move forward. Find new ways to contribute to the lives of the people you care about—there is always something that you can offer. Show yourself a little grace. You have a purpose and are valuable.

DAY 11:
The Chronic Pain Cycle

The sensation of pain is what happens in the brain after the nerves send out their signals (Day 2). But once that pain becomes chronic, a vicious cycle begins. The nervous system sets off alarm bells to warn us that something is wrong. This can cause us to grimace, grab the area, bend over to catch our breath, or cry out. In response, our muscles tighten and become tense. If those muscles remain tight for an extended period of time, inflammation will follow—our bodies are not designed to be in a constant state of stress. This then leads to fatigue and more pain.

When we experience pain and fatigue, our instinct is to rest and avoid anything that could make the discomfort worse—such as exercise or moving too quickly. This is beneficial while temporary, acute pain heals. However, for chronic pain, this actually contributes to the cycle. By remaining inactive, we often gain weight and our muscles become stiff and weak. This leads to poor posture and distorted motions, which create even more pain and can cause other injuries.

That would be difficult enough by itself, but it doesn't stop there. Chronic pain can also cause anger, irritability, guilt (Day 10), fear, frustration, and anxiety. Not being able to let go of these feelings will often lead to poor sleep, fatigue, and depression (Day 20)—all of which exacerbate the pain and can weaken the immune system.

Consider the following: You do not sleep well thanks to a sore neck. So you wake up stiff and exhausted, which increases your irritability and frustration. That stress causes your muscles to tighten even more, resulting in a surge of new pain. You stop exercising hoping it will heal, but that only weakens your muscles causing you to move differently—which creates yet more pain. Now imagine that neckache never gets better and the cycle continues to repeat itself day after day. The only way to stop it is to interrupt it.

- *Understand the cause.* Knowledge about your condition allows you to figure out what you need to change and why. It can give you the motivation and clarity to push forward.

- *Release muscle tension.* Trigger points or muscle knots are sensitive areas that remain tight even when the muscle is at rest. This knotted tissue needs to be relaxed in order to calm the inflamed nerves.

- *Treat the stiffness.* Gentle stretching keeps muscles flexible, strong, and healthy, and helps to improve posture, reduce stress, and maintain a proper range of motion in the joints. Heat is another tool that can be helpful in relieving stiffness. It works by increasing blood flow to the area to promote healing.

- *Stay hydrated.* It is no secret that water is

a basic necessity of life. It is essential for healthy muscles, tendons, joints, organs, and the very cells that make up our bodies. Even mild dehydration can have serious physical consequences. Yet eating and drinking with a chronic health condition can be challenging due to fatigue, loss of appetite, nausea, lack of mobility, or just feeling unwell.

- *Reduce the inflammation.* The cold from ice packs constricts blood vessels, which reduces swelling. Doctors often recommend alternating between ice and heat for the full benefit, since the first one reduces the inflammation and the other can reduce pain and promote healing. Many people find that compression clothing, such as socks or sleeves, also decreases pain and swelling. If you smash your finger, the first thing you might do is to grab it and apply pressure. This is instinctual and can ease the pain a little by disrupting the signals that are being sent to the brain. Compression garments can work the same way. Diet is also an important factor in reducing swelling. Certain foods are known to cause inflammation, while other foods can minimize it.

- *Stay active.* It is extremely difficult to get up and move when everything hurts and you are fatigued. However, our bodies were designed to be active. Movement is essential for maintaining flexibility, good blood circulation, and strength. It also improves our mood and reduces the risk of obesity and other health problems.

- *Replace negative thoughts*. The mind is a powerful tool, which is often underestimated and undertreated. Our thoughts and feelings can cause real physical symptoms. Think about something that makes you really nervous. Does it give you "butterflies" in your stomach or make you nauseous? Do your palms sweat, your muscles tense, or your voice shake? Does your face and neck turn red? These physical reactions are directly linked to your thoughts and emotions in that moment. When dealing with chronic pain, it is easy to give into toxic thoughts (Day 5).

Chronic pain is complex and needs to be treated according to each person's own unique situation. And while the things listed above are much easier said than done, they can help disrupt the pain cycle for many people.

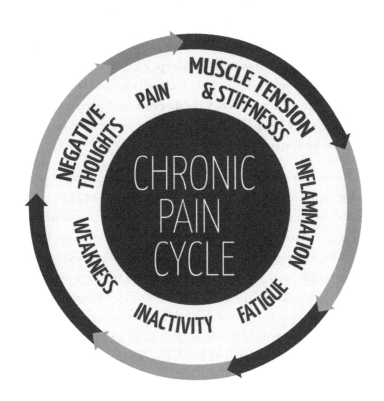

DAY 12:
Chronic Fatigue

Describing chronic, debilitating fatigue is a challenge and it is often misunderstood. Most people experience periods of low energy at some point in their lives. It may be caused by exertion, stress, lack of sleep, or an acute illness. It is normal to be overly tired or worn out after you have worked a 60-hour week, had a restless night of sleep, caught a virus, or are raising young kids. This fatigue is not extreme or persistent. It has a recognizable cause and generally goes away after getting enough rest or recovering from the illness.

On the other hand, chronic fatigue is something that you just cannot shake. It is an exhaustion that fills you to your core before you even begin any usual daily activities. Without any apparent reason, it sucks the energy right out of you. Your body feels weighted down—like you are trying to run uphill through mud after taking sleeping pills. Tasks that should ordinarily be easy become a struggle. It is so much more than being tired all the time. It is crippling, all-consuming, and not relieved by sleep. No matter how long you stay in bed, it never seems willing to release its hold on you. You often have a heightened sensitivity to sounds, smells, lights, or even touch—everything is tired, including your skin (Day 28). Yet, since the nature of fatigue is subjective, this symptom is often ignored by health care providers.

It can feel kind of like having the flu. Your muscles ache and are weak, it is hard to focus, you may feel dizzy, your limbs seem heavy, and you want to sleep until it is over. Some people even experience headaches, fever, or sore throat. On good days, it feels like you are just getting over the flu. Now you have enough energy to get up and do something, but you tire easily, struggle to concentrate, and still feel one step behind. You are a little stronger, but are constantly reminded that this gift comes with an expiration.

Imagine plugging in a dead cell phone before you go to bed at night. You expect it to be 100 percent charged when you wake up. However, most mornings it is at only 20 percent, and you have to function and make it through the day on that 20 percent. Sometimes you awake and are pleasantly surprised to find it at 30–40 percent, but it is never fully charged. This is what it is like to have chronic illness fatigue. Spoon theory has helped many people explain this concept to others (Day 8).

With chronic fatigue, you often compare yourself to other people your age who can work all day, go home to their kids, exercise, do household chores, and still have the energy for hobbies and friends. Then they get up the next day and do it all again. From the outside, their lives can seem so much more fulfilling than yours. They may even tell you, "I know what you mean. I feel tired all the time too." But the person who lives in your body uses almost every ounce of energy to get through the workday, somehow manages to make a piece of toast for dinner, and then leaves the dirty dishes in the sink because even the thought of washing them is too overwhelming. This person goes to bed early, but still wakes up the next morning feeling drained. Chronic fatigue is not just a fancy way of saying "really tired."

It can be helpful to remember that we only see what other people want us to see, especially on social media. We rarely know what actually goes on behind closed doors. When we convince ourselves that everyone else has it better, we start to ignore all the good in our own lives. However, the grass is often not greener on the other side of the fence. The grass is greenest wherever it is watered. So carry water along whatever path you find yourself on. When you stop comparing yourself to others and instead focus on growing what you have been given, you can begin to enjoy your unique journey more.

Living with chronic fatigue may mean that you have to change the way you see yourself. You are not the person with boundless energy who can do everything. And it is okay if you need to grieve that loss, even on a daily basis—it is not the ideal life, after all. It has ups and downs. While there will be times when you can barely lift your head off the pillow, there will also be periods when your symptoms ease up and you can do more. As a result, people with chronic fatigue have to be more intentional about their priorities, like saying no to a party in order to make it through their son's baseball game that night. Pacing is one of

the most important rules people with chronic illnesses need to learn (Day 27). Get rid of unrealistic
expectations. Instead of focusing on everything that
you cannot do, appreciate the things that you can do.
There will always be things that we cannot control, so
make the best of it, learn some lessons along the way,
and take each day as it comes.

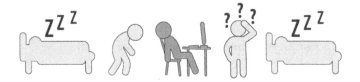

DAY 13:
Doctors Don't Know Everything

The medical world advances every day—from our understanding of how the body works to devices and medications that help us live longer. Most healthcare providers are amazing people who truly want to help. They are among the most highly trained professionals and have some of the most difficult jobs in the world. With that said, there is still so much that they do not know. They are only human after all.

Primary care physicians are expected to know a little bit about a lot of problems and do not specialize in one specific area. This makes it impossible for them to be familiar with every medical issue that exists, even some common ones. And with many new studies constantly being published—sometimes with conflicting information—it is simply unrealistic to expect every doctor to be up to date on all the latest research. This forces them to occasionally rely on outdated advice. If you suffer from chronic pain, you will probably find little comfort in the fact that this limited knowledge is frequently the reason why many healthcare providers fail to offer effective treatment.

On the other hand, patients do not need to know facts about thousands of different conditions. You only need to know about the ones that affect you. You can dedicate your time to issues that are most important to you personally and dig into research with single-minded focus. Finding journal articles and fully processing them takes a lot of time—as many chronic illness sufferers know all too well. You can also look into areas that doctors tend to shy away from professionally, like alternative medicine. And when it comes to conditions that are not widely known or understood, it often takes the desperate dedication of someone who has "skin in the game" in order to solve the mystery. No matter how much a doctor cares, it matters more to you.

A specialist is someone who focuses on one specific body system or symptom treatment, such as neurologists, cardiologists, or pain management. These doctors commit themselves to extra fellowships, additional tests, and extra hours of practice in their specialty. While their area of expertise is more concentrated than primary care physicians, that does not necessarily guarantee a less dismissive experience for a patient. Some sufferers finally get a specialist referral only to be told, once again, that their symptoms are all in their head or that they just need to deal with it. Being on the receiving end of this can be unbelievably frustrating and can lead to contentious doctor-patient relationships, incorrect diagnoses, prolonged suffering, or worsening symptoms. Even with all those years of training and hours of studying, it is impossible to know everything. The human body is incredibly complex (undeniably more complicated than any machine ever made) and sometimes symptoms simply do not fit perfectly into an expected model.

Besides limited knowledge, healthcare providers are also subject to bias. There is a saying in medicine that, "When you hear hoofbeats, think horses not zebras." This means that the provider should consider what is more common or likely. Doctors tend to dismiss side effects and symptoms they do not understand. They often err on the side of skepticism or disbelief when they cannot see something or detect it with tests. As a result, countless patients have been told that their very real symptoms are imaginary, unimportant, or coincidence—simply because they are outside the expected standard. But you know your body better than anyone else, and you know when something is wrong or off. When doctors do not experience chronic pain themselves, it can be hard for them to comprehend your situation. For years, many chronic illnesses were thought to be caused solely by depression or anxiety. The only treatment available for those patients was psychiatric care. Despite medical advances disproving this theory, some doctors are set in their ways. And for too many sufferers, ending up with physicians like this is commonplace. The fact is that sometimes the correct diagnosis is actually that proverbial zebra.

Self-reporting, although subjective, is currently the only way for a doctor to assess pain (Day 9). As a result, some medical practitioners downplay their patients' experiences. Those sufferers who refuse to accept their symptoms as normal or psychological are forced to read everything they can get their hands on and spend time searching for a doctor who understands their illness and offers appropriate treatment. All the while, their symptoms may be worsening or becoming more serious.

Therefore, it is important to educate yourself and seek advice from multiple experts. The better you understand and can describe your symptoms, the better equipped you will be to manage them and find help. With that said, there is no shortage of misinformation out there. At best, it is simply unhelpful. At worst, it is unhealthy and dangerous. Evaluate the sources carefully—not everything that looks official or trustworthy is credible. While it is not always the case, if an alternative cure or treatment sounds too good to be true, there is a good chance that it is. Also, it is important to recognize not only a doctor's biases in this area, but yours as well. Desperation can cloud a person's judgment, and there are many people out there who wish take advantage of that by offering false hope, which can be devasting. It also should be mentioned that once a patient has in-depth knowledge of their condition, they are more likely to encounter contempt from healthcare workers who do not like to be questioned. Once holes in their expertise are revealed, you may be considered difficult or non-compliant. At this point, you may need to look for a new physician. Being able to trust your provider, especially when you are at your most vulnerable, is essential and a fresh set of eyes can often be helpful.

Finding a healthcare professional who listens, investigates, advocates, and refers you to specialists who will work together with your regular physician is key. This is sometimes easier said than done, but is instrumental to receiving complete and proper care. While there are many understanding and compassionate doctors, some patients find nurse practitioners to be good listeners and more open to alternative treatment options, if that is what you are looking for. Other people have discovered that physical therapists can sometimes offer more personalized and targeted care. There is no one-size-fits-all approach. The goal is to find any medical professional who will take the time to carefully examine your needs and form the best treatment plan, regardless of whether or not they are a specialist.

DAY 14:
Brain Fog

Brain fog is common for people living with chronic pain and is extremely frustrating. Although it can be difficult to describe, many people use words like *forgetful* or *fuzzy-headed*. It is a cognitive dysfunction. Cognitive function includes a variety of mental activities such as memory, learning, problem solving, decision making, and attention. Therefore, someone who has brain fog may experience difficulty concentrating and processing information, confusion, or forgetfulness. You often know what you want to say, but just cannot find the thoughts or words to communicate effectively. It can feel like your head is stuffed full of mud. Trying to think straight becomes an impossible task and even things like coordination can be affected. Work, school, parenting, and other daily responsibilities become much more challenging when dealing with brain fog.

Most people know what it is like to lose your train of thought after you start saying something. But for many with chronic pain, this can be a common occurrence. If this is happening to you, you are not alone.

Brain fog itself is not a medical condition, but it can be a symptom of something else.

Depression and anxiety—Being sad or stressed out once in a while is completely normal. However, if you feel anxious, depressed, or hopeless for an extended period of time, it may become difficult to think clearly because these emotions steal your focus and are mentally exhausting. It is like trying to find one thought hidden somewhere in a dark cloud. As a result, people with depression often struggle to make decisions or complete daily tasks.

Lack of sleep—Insomnia is known to reduce mental sharpness and cognitive performance. When you do not get enough sleep, your brain cannot rest and recover. This means that it cannot function at its best when you are awake. Chronic fatigue (Day 12) is not only physically exhausting, but mentally draining as well. It can become difficult to have conversations because the words often seem to disappear before you can say them. There is no known cure for chronic fatigue, and it can leave the sufferer in a state of forgetfulness with an inability to focus.

Medications—Certain medications can leave you feeling foggy and patients are seldom warned about this possible side effect beforehand. Chemotherapy is a good example of this. *Chemo brain* is a common term used by patients to describe the thinking and memory problems that can occur during and after the treatment.

Pain—Chronic pain can interfere with cognitive functions, especially memory. A brain that is continually registering pain is over-activated and over-stressed, which can make it hard to focus. It can interfere with your concentration, as well as your ability to organize your thoughts. Fibromyalgia patients often call it *fibro fog*, but this cognitive dysfunction is common with many chronic illnesses.

If you are experiencing brain fog thanks to chronic pain, is there anything you can do?

Try clearing out some of the unwanted stimulation. Find a dim, quiet place to let your brain rest. Our cell phones, computers, and televisions cause our brains to work harder, so take a break from them for a bit. Distraction can also help reduce some of the background noise. This can include things like listening to music, journaling, or coloring. Exercise has also been shown to boost mental function and improve depression and anxiety.

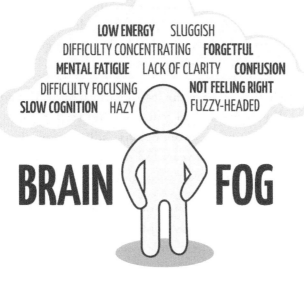

DAY 15:
Prevalence

Exact numbers are hard to find. As a result, data on the number of people living with chronic pain is far from complete, but anyone is at risk. It can come about with age or your genetics, as a result of surgery or an infection, from an injury or even some unknown cause. In 2011, chronic pain alone affected approximately 100 million Americans—more than the number of people with heart disease, diabetes, and cancer combined.[5] That is just over 30 percent of the population and has likely increased since then. And a report from The American Academy of Pain Medicine indicates that more than 1.5 billion people worldwide suffer from chronic pain.[6] It is an epidemic that is not getting the attention it deserves.

Chronic illnesses are the leading cause of death and disability in the United States and are responsible for seven out of every ten deaths—killing more than 1.7 million people a year. 133 million Americans have at least one chronic disease.[7]

Little research has been done to examine chronic pain trends, but a study published in 2021 found that the persistent and under-acknowledged pain problem continues to get noticeably worse.[8] During the study period of 2002–2018, they found that pain prevalence—already at a baseline high—increased substantially. This growth occurred in virtually all population subgroups, although adults at lower socioeconomic levels showed steeper pain increases.

People today are experiencing more pain than those in earlier decades. In fact, it seems that each generation is in greater pain at the same age than the one that came before it. It seems like all our medical advances should lead to a decline in pain, but the data strongly suggests the opposite.

Close to 11 million American adults have what is categorized as High-Impact Chronic Pain (HICP).[9] That is, pain lasting longer than three months and is accompanied by at least one major activity restriction—such as an inability to work outside the home, go to school, or perform household chores. People living with HICP report more severe pain, more mental health issues and cognitive impairments, and more difficulty caring for themselves than other chronic pain patients.

Chronic pain significantly impacts both the sufferer and those around them. Beyond just the patients and their families, it has consequences in social and professional environments as well in the health care system. Chronic pain is a major challenge confronting our modern culture. It ravages the lives of millions of families economically, physically, and emotionally. Yet chronic pain seems to fly under the radar when it comes to awareness and media attention.

CHORONIC PAIN

100 MILLION   🚹 = 1 MILLION

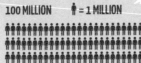

CHORONIC ILLNESS

133 MILLION   🚹 = 1 MILLION

DAY 16:
Gender

Chronic illness affects women and men differently, and women are more likely to experience it. Some health challenges that are unique to women are obvious, such as conditions that result from pregnancy or cancers of female reproductive organs. However, sometimes this is more nuanced. And while women are diagnosed with more nonfatal chronic illnesses, men are more likely to have fatal chronic conditions.

When it comes to smoking, women are two times more likely to develop lung cancer compared to men. However, women are roughly half as likely to die of the disease and respond better to chemotherapy.[10]

With a female-to-male ratio of 2.5:1, women are more than twice as likely to be diagnosed with irritable bowel syndrome (IBS).[11]

Nearly two-thirds of adults with Alzheimer's are female. The estimated lifetime risk at age 65 was 17 percent for women and 9 percent for men.[12] Even after factoring in women's typically longer lifespans, research suggests that sex-specific genes and crucial differences in the brain appear to be why women are at greater risk for this devastating disease.

Chronic pain is reported consistently higher in women than men, and women are at greater risk for many pain conditions. A paper by the National Academies of Sciences Engineering Medicine explained that women with cancer report greater pain severity and higher rates of depression than men. A number of chronic pain disorders occur only in women, while others occur predominantly in women—by as much as 80 to 90 percent. These include chronic fatigue syndrome, endometriosis, fibromyalgia, interstitial cystitis, vulvodynia, and temporomandibular disorders. In total, an estimated 50 million American women have one or more of these conditions. Furthermore, medication side effects and complications are also more common in women than men.[13]

Like many autoimmune conditions, multiple sclerosis (MS) is much more common in women than in men—by a ratio of 3:1. However, men tend to experience a more aggressive form of the disease compared to women.

Women are more than 2 times more likely to suffer from severe headaches or migraines. In the US, 17 percent of children between the ages of 4 and 18 experience frequent or severe headaches, including migraines. Before puberty, these occur in boys and girls at approximately the same rate. However, after the age of 12, the rate rises among girls.[14]

Why do these differences exist?

> - Women are more vulnerable to developing musculoskeletal pain. As they age, women experience more fractures, loss of bone mass, vertebral changes (such as

scoliosis), and arthritis. These things all cause joint pain, stiffness, and inflammation.

- Women are more likely to show signs of depression (Day 20). Depression is the most common women's mental health problem, and more women than men are diagnosed with depression each year. This can exacerbate pain and weaken the immune system.

- Almost 50 percent of women say that their stress levels are on the rise, compared to 39 percent of men. And women are more likely to show physical symptoms of stress, such as headaches, weakness, upset stomach, or indigestion.[15]

- Things like pregnancy, prescription birth control, and hormone replacement therapy can increase a person's risk of multiple ailments.

- Women are more likely than men to experience urinary tract problems. In fact, 40 percent of women will get a urinary tract infection (UTI) in their lifetimes while only 12 percent of men will get the same condition. This is due to the way the female urinary tract is structured.[16]

- Women are more likely to be impacted by pain after puberty, and many chronic conditions peak during the female reproductive years. This suggests a link between female sex hormones and the development of certain illnesses.

-    New studies are discovering a genetic basis for gender differences when it comes to certain conditions and chronic pain—like genes, genetic correlations, and patterns of tissue expression.[17]

2	LUNG CANCER	1	Chemotherapy less efffective and more likely to die
2	ALZHEIMER'S	1	
2.5	IBS	1	Current treatments less effective
3	MIGRAINES	1	
3	MS	1	More agressive form more likely

DAY 17:
Age

"You're too young to be on those medications or to be in pain like that." No one is too young for chronic pain. It does not discriminate and can affect people of all ages. It does not care how old you are. There is a commonly held belief that chronic illnesses are only for older people. However, the human body is incredibly complex and anything can go wrong, at any moment, and at any age.

Life as an adolescent or young adult is often difficult enough on its own, but those with chronic pain are frequently met with challenges beyond the usual suffering. Some physicians dismiss the symptoms simply because they are unwilling to look past the age listed on the chart. Yet living in daily pain can make you feel decades older than you actually are. As a result, many young people do not get the care that they desperately need.

It is not only healthcare workers who add to the struggle. Sometimes friends and family also have a difficult time understanding (Day 6). They would not expect an 80-year-old to have boundless energy or hang out every night, but they may not give the same courtesy to someone who is much younger. This is complicated further by the fact that chronic illness symptoms often ebb and flow. There are times when you may seem just like anyone else your age, but on other days you feel 80 years old and cannot even get out of bed. Instead of trying to understand, it is often easier to just think that person is lazy and making up excuses. After all, at their age, they should be able to bounce back, get over it, or sleep it off, right? But that is just not the case for everyone. When someone is repeatedly told that their condition cannot possibly be chronic, they feel ignored and may begin to question if what they are going through is even real (Day 19).

Then there are the extra personal challenges. When you are young, it is easy to forget that there are things that you cannot do—like lifting heavy objects, standing or sitting for too long, staying up late, or eating certain foods. Your peers often outpace you and you might try to keep up with them. It is not uncommon to overdo it and set yourself back (Day 27).

Children can also suffer from many of the same types of pain that adults experience, as well as chronic diseases that appear during childhood (like sickle-cell anemia, cystic fibrosis, or juvenile diabetes). As explained in the previous chapter, 17 percent of American children get frequent or severe headaches, including migraines. Additionally, conditions like asthma, hay fever, and ear infections occur more often in children and teens with recurrent headaches—42 percent compared to 25 percent in those without.[18] Yet children are often underdiagnosed, even when the headaches severely impact their lives. Once the pain is finally recognized, it is often undertreated. One of the main reasons for this is that prescribing pain medication for children is difficult. Most of these medications are not recommended for children and adolescents. Kids are not just small adults. Their bodies and brains are still developing.

When a condition is unexpected and believed to only occur in adults, such as endometriosis, young people are often left undiagnosed, untreated, and led to believe that their debilitating symptoms are normal.

Pain is usually considered an inevitable part of getting older. As we age, some physical wear and tear is natural. The cartilage that cushions our joints deteriorates, the discs in our spine lose fluid and become thinner, and our muscles become weaker. Postsurgical pain becomes more common, and there are conditions associated with aging, such as shingles. This creates an extra hurdle when you add chronic pain into the mix—which is extremely prevalent in older adults and is associated with limited mobility, social isolation, and depression. It becomes more difficult to distinguish between serious conditions and the natural process of getting older. This can result in warning signs being overlooked by both patients and physicians.

PAIN DOES NOT DISCRIMINATE BASED ON AGE.

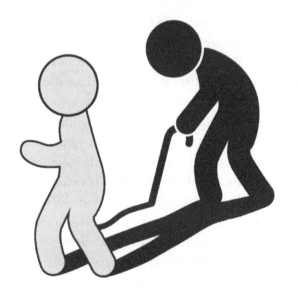

LOOKS
LIKE
VS.
FEELS
LIKE

DAY 18:
Alone

In addition to the physical and emotional discomfort, chronic pain can make you feel lonely—even if you know that you are not alone. You logically recognize that many others around the world are also struggling from the same illness, and you may even be surrounded by loving and empathetic friends and family. Yet in your daily life, you never seem to come across anyone who can truly relate. This can feel like you are all by yourself, even in a crowded room. As a result, chronic pain often isolates and separates us from others. We withdraw in an attempt to cope—distancing ourselves, even from those we love.

In order to move out of that isolation, you need to connect with others by sharing and opening up. However, it is often easier to just say that you are fine when someone asks how you are doing. We hide our pain in order to not cause our loved ones to worry more than they already do. We remain silent because we have been disbelieved too many times before (Days 19 and 24). We keep our struggles to ourselves because most people will never really understand, and in reality, they often do not want to know anyway. So we downplay our experience and keep the true depths of our pain to ourselves.

We do not want to be some version of Eeyore, the pessimistic and gloomy friend of Winnie the Pooh. Or like Moaning Myrtle, the easily distraught complainer from the Harry Potter series. In a world where independence, strength, and dependability are favorable qualities, there is a level of shame (Day 10) that comes with being sick all the time. Pain is seen as weakness, which for many translates into not being good enough. So we keep it inside in an effort to protect ourselves.

While opening up is necessary to escape the loneliness, it is easier said than done. Not only is there a possibility of rejection, but talking about the pain brings it to the forefront. The purpose of pain is to get our attention in order to warn us (Day 2). Yet people with chronic pain work so hard at trying to push it to the side in order to keep living life, and verbalizing the details of our symptoms brings us face to face with them. On the other hand, disconnecting from others and living in a bubble means that the pain has taken over our lives and controls our decisions—it has won. In reality, the pain will not go away by not talking about it, but the loneliness can.

It often seems like there is no one to talk to who will truly understand. The fact is that there are people who simply will not care or will hold it against you, and that makes it important to use wisdom in determining who to share your story with—although you may be surprised to discover that others are going through similar experiences that they have been hiding as well.

There can also be comfort in online communities of people who are fighting the same battle as you are.

Sometimes you just need to hear, "I get it and I've been there." You can find support from people you have never met because there is an instant understanding. Make an effort to connect with others.

Chronic illness can be lonely. Your body will continually betray you. People will call you lazy or dramatic. Others will offer unsolicited advice. You will miss out on things. But you are not alone.

DAY 19:
Not Crazy or Neurotic

"It's all in your head."

"You're being overly dramatic."

"What a crybaby."

"You're choosing to feel this way."

"That's all normal. There's nothing wrong with you."

Gaslighting is a form of manipulation that attempts to discredit someone by making them doubt their sanity, perception, or judgment. Having a chronic illness, especially an invisible one (Day 4), can make a person vulnerable to this tactic. It can come from family or friends who try to convince you that you are imagining it all or from healthcare professionals who disregard your symptoms (Day 13). This is so common that many chronic pain patients go into medical appointments expecting to not be believed. Pleading for someone to listen often becomes a regular part of the journey.

The average length of time for someone to receive a postural tachycardia syndrome (POTS) diagnosis is almost six years. And 69 percent of POTS patients are initially told their symptoms are just anxiety.[19] It takes an average of six years and four different physicians for someone with lupus to be properly diagnosed, and it too is often mistaken for an anxiety disorder.[20] For endometriosis it is seven to nine years[21], often because patients are repeatedly told their symptoms are completely normal. Yet it is estimated that 1 in 10 women have it. Many other examples could be cited, but the point is that medical gaslighting is not uncommon.

To be fair, it is far more complex than it may appear. First, primary care doctors are not specialists, which can make it difficult for them to recognize symptoms (Day 13). In addition, specialists can sometimes be so siloed into their area of expertise that if a symptom list does not fit perfectly into a condition, they disregard the patient's complaints. Second, the link between anxiety and chronic pain can be a diagnostic challenge. Many people do have anxiety. Palpitations, dizziness, chest pain, headaches, nausea, and abdominal cramps can all be symptoms of anxiety—but they can also be symptoms of other conditions. And then there is cause and effect. Are chronic illness symptoms making the patient anxious, or is anxiety causing the symptoms? Ignoring someone's symptoms or questioning their sanity is not helpful in answering that question. Medical gaslighting leads to sick people not getting the correct testing or not being referred to appropriate specialists. And it means that they will not receive the necessary treatments.

Imposter syndrome is defined as "a collection of feelings of inadequacy that persist despite evident success." This is especially common among high-achieving individuals. They feel like frauds—like their successes are because of luck and not their own skill.

Medical imposter syndrome is becoming more recognized. When you go through years of normal test results and multiple doctors telling you that nothing is wrong, you can begin to feel like a phony. You start to question whether or not your symptoms are even real and you begin to accept the labels: *whiner, crazy, hypochondriac*. Then when you finally achieve success in your medical journey by receiving a diagnosis, you might still doubt yourself. After years of absorbing words of dismissal, they become a part of you. It is difficult to just stop feeling like a fraud in your own body.

You can especially feel like an imposter when your symptoms ebb and flow. On good days, it is easy to forget why you maintain a strict diet, take medication, or are incapable of working. Maybe you are not really that sick after all? Good days bring false hope. If your symptoms are barely noticeable today, maybe they will be completely gone tomorrow—maybe forever. Imposter syndrome urges you to push yourself beyond your known limitations. It is difficult to not overdo it on good days (Day 27), but your illness is always there, waiting to remind you that it is not going anywhere.

Even after a valid diagnosis, it is easy to question any new or worsening symptoms. *Am I being extra sensitive? Maybe I am a hypochondriac? Am I imagining it? Maybe I should just ignore it? Should I go to the emergency room or call my doctor? Will they roll their eyes at me again?* These kinds of thoughts can cause you to try to push through your body's warning signs, which in turn can make the symptoms even worse. Because pain is an individual and subjective experience, you need to be able to trust yourself when something is not right.

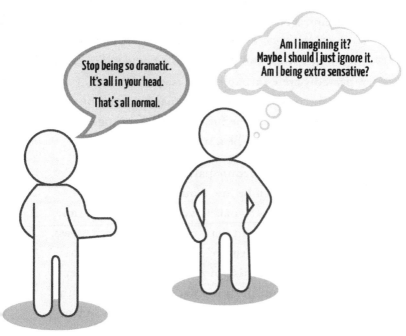

DAY 20:
Depression and Suicide

Chronic illnesses can have a negative effect on a person's self-worth (Day 7). It is natural to feel sad or discouraged after receiving a diagnosis. You may go through stages of grief (denial, anger, bargaining, depression, and acceptance). Some people even repeatedly cycle through these stages. After all, you are facing new limitations and may be afraid of the treatments or what the future holds. Coping with your new reality can be a struggle.

When you are in chronic pain, your threshold for other burdens can be low. Your body is continually sending stress signals to your brain, which can trigger depression, anxiety, or post-traumatic stress disorder (PTSD). Prolonged pain can cause emotional distress. At this point, it begins to take over every area of your life and affects your ability to find happiness in anything. It is demoralizing as well as physically and emotionally draining, which often makes the pain even worse (Day 11). Breaking this vicious cycle is difficult.

In addition, some conditions actually change the brain, which can play a direct role in depression. And the side effects of certain medications can trigger it. Worrying about higher medical costs or watching healthy peers enjoy more experiences can also affect your mental health. Long-lasting stress and anxiety can upset the immune, digestive, and reproductive systems. It can increase the risk of heart attack, stroke, and other serious health problems. The fact is that any chronic condition can trigger depression, but the risk increases with the severity and the level of life disruption it causes. And depression often intensifies pain, fatigue (Day12), and brain fog (Day 14).

Opening up about depression is personal and emotional. However, not talking about it isolates you and makes you feel alone (Day 18). The more often that people tell you to "just be positive" or "just don't think about the pain," the more disconnected you can become. You start to wonder how much longer you can live like this, and you long for the pain to end.

Depression affects each person differently, and sometimes the symptoms are masked by other ailments. But it is a common complication of chronic illness. It is estimated that up to one-third of people living with a chronic condition have symptoms of depression,[22] and depressed patients are less likely to follow their treatment plans—which then results in poorer health and worse pain. However, it does not have to be an inevitable part of your journey. There is no one-size-fits-all treatment, and it may take some trial and error to find the best approach for you.

As illness takes away different aspects of life, it can be a struggle to move forward. In 2016, suicide was the 10th leading cause of death across all ages.[23] Several large-scale studies have shown that at least 1 in 10 suicides are linked to chronic illness or unrelenting pain, and nearly all physical health conditions are associated with increased suicide risk. The true number of failed attempts is unknown and may never be determined, but one study found that roughly 50 percent of chronic pain patients reported having seriously considered suicide as a way to end the suffering.[24] High-risk characteristics include being younger than 45 years old, female, unemployed, or divorced. Other pertinent factors include alcohol dependence, past suicide attempts, and poor social support systems.

Being in constant pain is horrible. If you get your symptoms under control, it can help improve the signs of depression as well. When the depression is a side effect of your medications, adjusting them or choosing a different treatment plan may help—which both should be done under the guidance of your physician. There are also medications that are designed to treat depression. And as explained on Day 5, cognitive behavioral therapy (CBT) can help some people develop skills to better cope with the symptoms.

Do you view yourself as a victim losing the battle or a fighter who will never give up? When all you have in your day is pain, it can be difficult to find joy in anything. Accept that life is different, forgive your body and yourself, and realize that you are not alone.

DAY 21:
Employment and Disability

Having a chronic illness shakes up your world. Unless you were born with your condition, you went from being healthy and enjoying life to struggling to finish simple daily tasks. Things that used to be easy now require careful planning. Spoon Theory (Day 8) explains how just getting out of bed, making a meal, or showering can use up precious limited energy. While other people are working full-time, taking care of their families, and still finding time for social activities, your main concern now is making it through each day before your battery is completely drained (Day 12). You have to budget your energy in order to figure out how many things you can get done before your body crashes (Day 27). But sometimes it is impossible to balance that budget. Pushing your limits is often seen as a way to better yourself and reach your goals, but for chronic illness sufferers, that can have serious negative effects on your health.

There are laws to help protect employees from being fired due to a disability, but the reality is that at some point your work is going to suffer. On average, American workers miss 4.6 hours a week due to chronic pain.[25] However, the majority of lost productivity is in the form of reduced work performance instead of absences.

Chronic illnesses can be unpredictable. Between symptoms, medications, and doctors' appointments, your productivity frequently varies and your abilities can change on a daily or even hourly basis. It is easier to balance a budget when you have a good idea what your salary will be every month. Now imagine being a freelancer. Managing finances with this type of income becomes more of a challenge because there is little certainty or consistency. That is what it is like working with a chronic illness. You need to regularly budget your energy without knowing how much you will have from one day to the next.

Since our culture values reliability and maximum efficiency, having a job can leave you with an incredibly difficult choice—a paycheck or your health. It can be a real challenge to stay employed and take good care of yourself at the same time. Yet many chronically ill employees need to continue working to keep their health insurance in order to help cover the financial burden (Day 3) of the seemingly never-ending medical bills.

When you have an invisible illness (Day 4), you may find that your boss or colleagues doubt the severity of your condition. You can also become a target if your co-workers feel like you are unfairly receiving special accommodations.

If you reach a point where it becomes impossible to work, even on a part-time basis, you will probably start to look into disability. As of the writing of this book, applications for pain-related disability are at an all-time high. But you may find that your doctors—the same ones who diagnosed and are treating you—will not sign off on any forms. Many offices have policies now that prevent them from filling out disability paperwork. Even specialists often refuse and send the patients back to their primary care office because they feel that the liability is too high for those who are faking it. You might hear something similar to what numerous others have been told, "Yes, chronic migraines are considered a disability. But it's a very long and difficult process, so we don't do that here." You can have a debilitating illness, be medically disabled, and still be denied benefits.

People who are unable to work due to chronic illness are not "on vacation" or "so lucky." They do not have "unlimited free time." Their time is spent being sick and trying to make it through basic daily activities. Many sufferers would rather be at work—that would mean that they are healthy enough. Between the physical and emotional symptoms, doctor and therapy appointments, record keeping, medication schedules, tests, procedures, and the day-to-day uncertainty (Day 23), being chronically ill can feel like a full-time job in itself.

DAY 22:
Changes Everything

Living with a chronic illness changes how you use your time and energy (Day 8), what jobs—if any—you are able to do (Day 21), how much help you require throughout the day, and every relationship that you have. The pain and fatigue become just a regular part of everyday life. Regardless of the condition's name, the struggle to adjust is real.

No matter how tempted you are to deny or ignore it, this is your new life—your new normal. It requires you to rethink everything and set reasonable expectations for yourself. You may experience grief, which is a natural response to loss. This might include the loss of independence, income, comfort, mobility, relationships, spontaneity, control, or just the person who you were before. It is okay to feel different now because you are different. Change is part of the process.

Self-care cannot wait for you to find the time anymore. It has become mandatory. Feeling independent is a thing of the past. There will be times when it is necessary to ask for help, accept support (Day 29), and embrace the generosity of others. You have to learn how to advocate for yourself with doctors, with your employer, and with family and friends.

Everyone's life is full of tough choices, but those choices change once chronic illness takes control. Do you skip a meal and get sick and fatigued or eat and get sick and nauseous? Are alternative and unconventional treatments worth the financial (Day 3) and physical risk? Do you use your limited energy to go to your son's basketball game or your daughter's dance recital? Do you push your body to its limit and pay for it over the next few days or play it safe to see what tomorrow brings (Day 27)? Should you spend your energy taking a shower or just get by without one— again (Day 8)? Do you keep your health issues private and risk people thinking you are lazy or talk openly and risk people thinking that you are crazy (Day 19)? Do you ignore a new symptom because you might be overreacting or go see your doctor because it might be serious? Should you aggressively fight to regain your health or just accept things the way they are?

To healthy people, things like showering, making a meal, or doing the dishes may seem like routine or easy or choices, but they can have a big impact on the daily life of someone with a chronic illness. There are many considerations to keep in mind. Can you physically finish the task? Will you need help? Do you have enough energy? Will it make you unable to complete, or even start, an important future task? Making the right decision is important, but not as easy as it may seem. When you see someone who is battling a chronic illness, keep in mind that they have made a lot of small yet difficult choices to get to where they are. And many of those decisions are ones that most people take for granted and never give much thought to.

Simply getting dressed can be complicated. Besides the energy that it takes, you may not be able to simply throw on whatever clothes you want. What can you physically put on that day? If your hands are hurting, buttons are out of the question. But if you cannot lift your arms, that also rules out pullover shirts. Can you wear pants and what kind? Leggings or jeans might seem comfortable at the moment, but they will become incredibly painful if you bloat later. Do you have bruises or a brace that you want to keep covered? Pants and long sleeves, even on a hot day, will be your only option then. Do you suffer with temperature irregularities? Make sure you have layers that can easily be removed and put back on. Is your skin feeling overly sensitive? Well, certain materials or styles will be itchy or painful.

Learning to adjust to all the changes and cope with new limitations can be difficult. Life is different than what it once was and not at all what you expected it to be. But you can go on, reshape your priorities, and grow where you have been planted.

DAY 23:
The Unknown

What are your plans for 10 years from now? What about five years? How about tomorrow? For many people with a chronic illness, it is almost impossible to answer with more than, "It depends how I feel." While it is natural to want some stability in life, your condition is just too unpredictable.

The uncertainty of each day presents a unique challenge. It is difficult to forecast how you will feel at any given point—and there is not much you can do about it. It is like exploring uncharted land. You may start the day on beautiful flat ground but end up climbing a mountain. The next morning you find yourself trekking through knee-high mud, which then turns into a smooth and easy patch. Or the entire day could be spent walking through thorns or along a beach. Every day is an adventure and you never know what to expect. When you are living with a chronic illness, the path is not always straight and scenic.

This can be confusing to outsiders who see someone upbeat and ready to take on the world one day and then looking like a mess and barely able to move the next. Sometimes the symptoms are manageable—giving the sufferer a much-needed respite—and this can make it appear as if they are faking during the bad times. In reality, they are simply trying to take advantage of what their body will allow in the moment.

However, even on the good days, you are trying to brace yourself and prepare for the worst. Imagine sitting in a boat on the ocean. The water is calm and quiet at the moment, but your eyes search the sky for the impending storm. It is not a matter of if but when the turbulence will return. You also must continually check the water on all sides. It looks clear for now, but there are hidden dangers lurking below—predators whose only goal is to knock you off the boat when you least expect it. It might be today, tomorrow, or a week from now, but it is going to happen. In this situation, it would be quite difficult to fully enjoy the fresh air and beauty all around you, the warm sun kissing your skin, and the pod of playful dolphins in the distance. This is what it is like living every day in the unknown of chronic illness.

Life itself can be unpredictable enough, but there is even more uncertainty about the future when you add a chronic illness into the mix. *Will I ever get better or will I continue to get worse? How will I support myself if I can't work? Will people understand and accept me? Will I die from this condition?* These types of questions are normal, yet you have little to no control over the answers.

After every new medication, treatment, or surgery, it is easy to hope that you can finally put the pain behind you and start fresh. Maybe this is the thing that is going to cure you. Maybe it is the answer you have been looking for. But then the harsh reality grabs ahold of you and reminds you yet again that your constant companion is not going anywhere.

There may be times when something comes along and offers you some relief. It works so well that you start to let down your guard and dare to dream about a pain-free future. Then, seemingly out of nowhere, your body betrays you again and demands a new and stronger treatment. If you get your hopes up, they will usually get crushed. But you also do not want to spend your life always assuming the worst. It is a fine line to tread.

Recognize that you are not choosing this; your body is choosing it for you and it does not care if you made plans or not. Just because your illness is invisible (Day 4) does not make it any less debilitating at times. The fact is that there will always be far more questions than answers, and there are no simple solutions. You may never be able to solve all the mysteries, find a cure, or simply make definite plans. But as long as you still have a heartbeat, you can keep searching and fighting—one breath at a time.

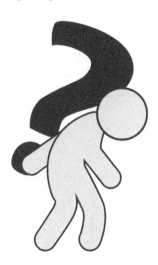

DAY 24:
Can't Judge a Book by the Cover

This has been mentioned multiple times throughout this book, but it deserves its own chapter. We all judge books by their covers—that is natural. Our minds attempt to fill in the blanks with information that we do not have yet. We are unlikely to even look at the description on the back of a book if the front is unappealing. How many people start reading a terrible story just because the cover was beautiful? We may even ignore glaring red flags because of a tempting outward appearance. And no matter how hard we try to fight it, we still do it now and then.

It is time to make a conscious effort to go against that natural instinct. People have stories too. They have experiences that make them who they are. Our preconceived ideas about how they look can deceive us into making incorrect assumptions. The reality is that everything is not always as it seems and external appearances can be manipulated. Multiple people have been credited with saying, "Your assumptions are your windows on the world. Scrub them off every once in a while, or the light won't come in."

"But you don't look sick."

"You look (or sound) too good for someone who has your condition."

These types of statements may or may not be said

with malice. But no matter the intent, they give rise to the idea that the person is not truly very ill and are dismissive of the symptoms and pain. This can be a hurdle when talking to others about your health and diagnosis. We are visual beings and people with chronic illnesses are usually portrayed as looking run down and messy, bedridden, with pale or splotchy skin, moving slowly with a cane, or just simply having an overall unwell appearance. In reality, you do look like that sometimes, or a lot of the time, but most people do not see you during the hard periods. On the good days, you attempt—often at great cost—to get out of the house. And when you do, you try your best to blend in and look normal. People often form their opinions around these moments, so when they see you out smiling and having fun, they think that you are either all better or were making the whole thing up. Instead, you are simply trying to live as opposed to just existing.

The general public has a difficult time believing that someone is in pain or has a major health issue when their looks say otherwise. The assumption is that if a person appears normal, then they are capable of doing normal things—and that can be incorrect. People who do not live with a chronic, life-changing condition will never completely understand the effort it takes to try to blend in, and yet attempting to do so can help the sufferer feel human again. So instead of "faking being sick," you have to become a master at "faking being well."

Faking wellness is a double-edged sword. On one hand, you do not want to look sick. And for those who do not want to talk about their illness, this allows them to temporarily blend in with society. But on the other hand, you also want people to know what you are going through and to not falsely judge you. You would like people to understand that even though your illness and pain are invisible (Day 4), they are always a struggle.

When you hear the dreaded, "But you don't look sick," you feel like people do not believe you. They cannot see the strength it took to stand up and leave your house. They cannot feel the pain raging through your body. They cannot understand the effort that is required to force yourself to do simple tasks. So change your perspective and take it as a compliment from now on. It means that your smile is believable and more powerful than the pain. It means that you did an amazing job of getting dressed and looking presentable. It means that you are tougher than most people will ever know. It means that you are standing up to something that would knock most people to the floor. It means that you are a fighter and did not let the pain win that day. That makes you more than a survivor; you are a conqueror.

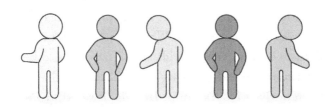

WHICH ONE HAS A CHRONIC ILLNESS?

DAY 25:
Opioid Crisis

Opioids are a class of drugs used to block pain signals between the brain and body. They can be prescription pain relievers, such as oxycodone and Vicodin, or so-called street drugs like heroin. Besides controlling pain, opioids are also known to make some people feel relaxed, happy, or high. Using these drugs on a regular basis can increase your tolerance and dependency, requiring higher and more frequent doses, which often leads to addiction. The definition of *narcotic* can get a little murky because it varies among agencies. While some say that cannabis, cocaine, and opioids are all narcotics, others maintain that narcotics are only substances that have been derived from opium. In today's world, the word *narcotics* has a negative connotation and is often more closely associated with illegal drugs. As a result, most medical professionals no longer use that term—even though all opioids are technically narcotics. The preferred term these days is *controlled substances*.

Historically, doctors emphasized pain management, which resulted in an overprescribing of opioids. In 2000, shortly before the pain scale (Day 9) became standardized and widely used, 126 million prescriptions for opioids were in circulation in the United States. By 2011, that number had risen to 219 million.[26] Prescription drugs are the second-most abused category of drugs in the United States, and overdose deaths involving opioids increased 519 percent from 1999 to 2019. Each year, prescription opioid abuse costs $78.5 billion in healthcare costs, legal programs, and lost productivity. The opioid epidemic is considered by many to be a public health emergency, with 136 deaths per day, a figure that continues to climb.[27]

There is no debate that narcotics can be dangerous when used incorrectly or illegally. However, there is another side to this crisis—one that rarely enters the conversation and does not get much media coverage. And it is affecting the treatment plans, quality of life, and ability to function for many chronic pain patients. The majority of doctors have either cut back on or stopped prescribing opioids all together. Medicare has restricted its supply, and the Drug Enforcement Agency (DEA) has decreased the amount produced. Also, some pharmacies have limited the opioid prescriptions they will fill.

While many believe that this is a logical response to the increased abuse, they are usually not the ones living with severe chronic pain that has yet to respond to any other treatment. As a result, those using opioids responsibly have been caught in the crossfire. When it comes to prescriptions, the rate of addiction averages between 8–12 percent.[28] That leaves an estimated 88–92 percent who were using them correctly.

So what does this crisis look like from the other side?

> - Having to make your very limited supply last because you may not be able to get

any more with all the new restrictions—restrictions that were not created because of your irresponsibility.

- Hoping to find a doctor who is not only well-versed in chronic pain, but who is also willing to acknowledge its disabling impact. Many pain management clinics have also adopted non-opioid treatment policies, so even seeing a pain specialist nowadays will get many of these patients nowhere.

- Choosing between being able to function during the day or being able to sleep at night since you do not have enough medication to do both.

- Being viewed as a "drug seeker" if your pain forces you into the emergency room. Often in these situations, the more you try to advocate for yourself, the more suspicion and resistance you are met with.

- Dealing with the consequences of other people's actions since you have never abused your opioids or purchased them illegally.

- Resorting to other, sometimes more dangerous options, to find a way to alleviate the pain.

Most people do not want narcotics, are aware of the risks, and would love to find something else that would relieve their pain as effectively. Currently not every condition has another treatment option though. Nobody should be shamed or have to live in disabling pain when there are medications that can help. However, there are strict laws for a reason and these powerful drugs should not be easily available to everyone. It is important to address the dangers and work toward preventing abuse. This is a dilemma in the fight against opioids, but people with chronic pain should not be ignored or viewed as merely collateral damage.

DAY 26:
Lifestyle

Your day-to-day life plays a key role in managing pain. For many chronic illness patients, learning to slow down is one of the most difficult skills to develop. You cannot do everything and that is a constant battle (Day 27). It is hard to feel left out when your body tells you to stay home. And while you spend so much time at home, you still are not able to complete all the household tasks that healthy people do. It is discouraging to break your day up into a hundred little jobs and then leave most of them unfinished because they are impossible to complete. This can leave you feeling unmotivated, even on days when you do have a little more energy.

Your lifestyle revolves around getting enough rest, yet too much physical inactivity can lead to more pain and worsened symptoms (Day 11). While there is a legitimate fear of wearing yourself out or causing more discomfort, staying sedentary has its own negative consequences. Your muscles lose endurance and strength. Your bones can also become weaker. The supply of blood and oxygen decreases throughout the body. Mental processing slows and blood pressure rises. You may gain weight, which can increase inflammation. You have a higher risk of developing diabetes, heart disease, and other serious conditions. Overall, being inactive—whether you have chronic pain or not—is not beneficial. There are going to be days when just getting out of bed is difficult, but even small activities or low-impact exercises can help your overall wellbeing and prevent future pain.

The mind and body are inherently connected (Day 5). Pain causes stress, and stress causes more pain. It is important to identify your stress triggers and work to reduce them. Even in times when the pain is minimal, you may have anxiety about when the suffering will return (Day 23). This can be crippling and detrimental to your quality of life.

Improving your sleeping habits can help reduce fatigue and mental distress. While the total number of hours is important, it is also necessary to get good-quality sleep. People who get enough rest tend to deal with their pain better than those who do not. However, that is not always easy to do. Pain is a thief that takes many things, but it loves to steal sleep. It becomes a vicious cycle. Pain keeps waking you up and in return, the lack of sleep makes the pain worse. Strategies for improving sleep include a cool bedroom (around 65 degrees), no digital devices in the room, a consistent sleep schedule, a clean bedroom, exercise, and a diet of foods that promote sleep. It is also possible to have an underlying sleep disorder. If this is the case, a sleep specialist can recommend a treatment plan that can help significantly.

Eat a healthy diet. Some chronic pain improves with weight loss because extra weight raises blood pressure, increases inflammation, and adds stress to the joints. Certain foods can also help fight or cause inflammation. Many patients find that changing their diet reduces pain and improves energy levels. Food sensitivities can also explain worsening symptoms when some people eat certain foods, despite them being part of the standard recommended healthy diet. In addition, things like pain, nausea, and fatigue can affect your eating habits. When you are not feeling well, eating is often the last thing on your mind.

Keep a pain diary. This is a daily record detailing your symptom levels, activities, and perhaps your diet. While this may be the last thing you want to spend your limited energy on, it can be a useful tool on your journey. It can be shown to doctors or therapists to help them understand the intensity and duration of your pain. It tracks how well medication is working or not working, and any side effects. It can give a clear picture of how specific activities or foods affect your pain. And sometimes these records are beneficial for insurance or legal purposes.

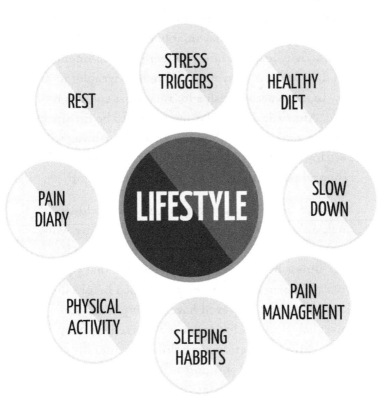

DAY 27:
Pacing and Post-Exertional Malaise

One of the most important rules for chronic illnesses is pacing. It can be quite difficult to balance activity and rest. It is often necessary to take breaks before they become unavoidable rather than basing your activity level on how you feel in the moment. On days when your symptoms are manageable, it is easy to try to accomplish a lot in a short amount of time. After all, day-to-day tasks need to be finished, and you never know when the next opportunity will be. However, pushing yourself can cause fatigue, rebound pain, and increased use of medication.

You wake up feeling pretty good, so you decide to catch up on as many things as possible. Failure will not be an option—this is war and you refuse to let your illness beat you today. The result is that you work all morning only to end up in bed before the day is over. You may even have accomplished some of your goals, but at what expense? Worsening symptoms, extra medication, irritability, or literally collapsing in pain? At this point, it may take you days or weeks to recover, and over time, you will be able to do less and less. Recovery is a slow process and there is no cheating.

Eventually, your symptoms settle down and you have another good day. If you did not learn your lesson, the pattern is repeated all over again. There is no one-size-fits-all strategy and pacing is not about giving up everything you want to do. The goal is to be as active as possible without experiencing post-exertional malaise (PEM), but the approach must be customized to each individual. Finding a balance between your desired activities and keeping flare-ups at bay is almost an art form, which can take time to develop.

Imagine driving your car until the gas light illuminates its one and only warning. *Empty*. At this point you have two choices. You can take the safe route and stop for gas right away or keep going because you know that there is a little bit left in the tank. If you decide to risk it, your car will eventually stop and become unmovable. It does not matter how hard you try or how positive your thinking is, the car is simply not going to go anywhere. Every chronic illness sufferer needs to learn their own limits in order to stop and refuel before they run completely dry. If you try to push through in order to make it just a little farther, the fumes run out and you have nothing left.

This is why pacing—and not using your pain as a guide—is necessary in order to break the cycle. Every activity has a price so create reasonable preset goals. For example, maybe you need a 10-minute break for every 20 minutes of activity. This can be tricky because it can change from day to day and things that you easily tolerated in the past may now be off limits. Determine your own individual boundaries, and then plan your activities and rest accordingly. The idea is to constantly be aware, adjust when necessary, and never fully hit your breaking point. Flare-ups will happen, but pacing can help limit them.

PEM is perhaps one of the most difficult things for many people to understand. It occurs when symptoms get worse following even minor physical or mental exertion, sometimes 12–48 hours later, and it can last for days or weeks. For healthy people, getting a little exercise is known to increase energy, improve mental sharpness, and can also decrease pain. However, for someone who experiences PEM, the result is the opposite. Physical, mental, or emotional tasks or social activities can be draining and lead to delayed but severe fatigue (Day 12), brain fog (Day 14), weakness, pain, headaches, and other symptoms.

Any activity or exercise plan needs to be individually based. Cleaning, preparing a meal, grocery shopping, or getting showered and dressed may need to be broken down into shorter, less strenuous pieces. For some people, even talking on the phone, sitting at a computer, or riding in a vehicle while someone else drives can lower energy to the point of exhaustion. While Spoon Theory (Day 8) is helpful in explaining this, it can be incredibly difficult to comprehend for anyone who has not experienced it.

Words like *crash*, *relapse*, *hangover*, or *collapse* are often used to describe PEM. It can be like having a bad flu or mononucleosis (mono). It feels almost impossible to get out of bed, walk to the bathroom, or even watch TV. You are exhausted to your very core. This can be mitigated by pacing, and the goal is to avoid PEM flare-ups and illness relapses.

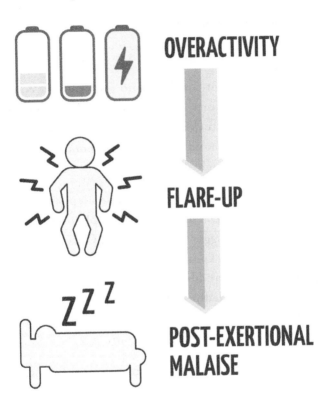

OVERACTIVITY

FLARE-UP

POST-EXERTIONAL MALAISE

DAY 28:
Hypersensitivity

"Even my hair hurts."

"Please turn that down."

"It's way too bright in here."

Sensitivity to light, smell, sound, or touch are common symptoms for chronic illnesses. When your immune system is stuck in high gear, constantly trying to fight off your condition, every system in your body seems to be on high alert.

For numerous conditions—such as epilepsy, fibromyalgia, and headache disorders—light plays a significant role as a trigger or a symptom. Chronic light sensitivity is also known as *photophobia*. It can cause pain in the eyes and brain as well as triggering dizziness, lightheadedness, headaches, blurred vision, and other symptoms. Sometimes it only requires a few seconds or minutes of exposure.

Blue light has been shown to be the most harmful in prompting or worsening symptoms, and it can be found almost everywhere—from fluorescent lighting to screens on electronic devices to sunlight. Intensity and movement can also be factors. For example, bright lights in stores and flashing or flickering lights can often cause nausea and magnify the other hallmark symptoms.

Although loss of smell (*hyposmia*) is more common in chronic illnesses, the opposite affect can also occur. *Hyperosmia* is a heightened and hypersensitive sense of smell. This lowers a person's threshold for odors and has been associated with conditions like migraines, Lyme disease, lupus, and multiple sclerosis (MS). Sensitivity to smells is not uncommon, especially during pregnancy or while taking some medications. People with hyperosmia can experience nausea, disgust, allergies, or migraines in response to certain smells. Individual irritants vary from person to person. While exposure to chemical odors like perfumes or cleaning products can trigger symptoms, even milder scents in things like shampoo or laundry detergent can also be too much.

A loud noise, especially when it is unexpected, can be jarring for anyone. But, *hyperacusis* is the name for an intolerance to sounds that would not bother most people. Everyday noises such as talking to a friend, watching TV, driving, or vacuuming can cause significant distress and make it difficult to deal with day-to-day activities. For people with hyperacusis, the ears detect the same sounds that everyone else hears, but the brain reacts differently and exaggerates the vibrations. As a result, the brain interprets each tiny noise as a direct assault. The world's volume seems unbearably high, which may cause physical pain or pressure in the ear. Some people even find their own voice to be intolerably loud. This can become overwhelming and lead to *phonophobia*, a fear of loud noises. Noise sensitivity is a symptom of numerous conditions such as migraines, nerve dysfunction, and some autoimmune disorders. Common symptoms include hearing loss, headache, dizziness, nausea, and unsteadiness.

Allodynia is a hypersensitive reaction to touch. It is often associated with fibromyalgia, migraines, and nerve disorders. This is pain, generally on the skin, that is caused by something that should not normally hurt—such as slight touch, vibration, heat, cold, or pressure. For example, taking a shower may seem like a basic, harmless activity, but it can present major problems for people with allodynia. Between the temperature change and the water hitting your skin, your nerves can get all riled up.

There are three different forms of allodynia:

1. Tactile or Static Allodynia: This is pain caused by pressure of something against your skin. It can hurt to wear glasses, rest your head on a pillow, get a hug, or wear clothing—especially the tighter parts like waistbands or bra straps.

2. Mechanical or Dynamic Allodynia: This type of pain is caused by movement across the skin. Triggers can be things like someone rubbing your arm, brushing your hair, water falling on you in the shower, or even the air from a fan blowing across your skin.

3. Thermal Allodynia: This is temperature-related pain caused by a mild change of temperature on the skin. For example, a few drops of warm water on the skin or breathing in cooler air may be painful.

Allodynia is not the same as *hyperalgesia*, which is an abnormally heightened sensitivity to painful stimuli. That is extreme pain caused by something minor, such as a paper cut or a small bruise. It essentially "turns up the volume" on pain. However, individuals with allodynia feel pain when something is ordinarily painless.

LIFE WITH HYPERSENSITIVITY

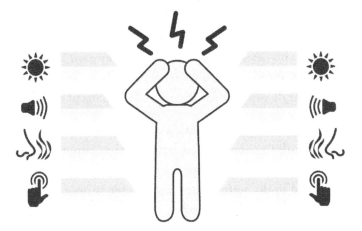

DAY 29:
Support

Sometimes it seems like nobody cares about your chronic illness. It can be discouraging to feel like you are being overlooked or not taken seriously, even when you can barely get out of bed. Try to remember that life is hard for everyone. You may not know what others are truly dealing with, just like they may not fully understand your struggles. The "Don't Judge a Book by Its Cover" mantra (Day 24) does not only apply to other people. The world can be a rough and unfair place, and sometimes people deal with their own hardships by trying to shut out the other bad things going on around them—including the challenges of others.

People often do want to help—temporarily. When someone is first diagnosed with cancer, loses their job, is recovering from surgery, or has a death in the family, many people will bring meals, send cards or money, and offer to help in any way they can. However, it is more difficult to expect people to keep up that level of support for the rest of the patient's life.

If you have a loved one with a chronic illness, it can be difficult to show endless patience, but support is everything. People who have a strong support system tend to do better long-term. Since support is so valuable, what can you do?

Ask yourself how you would want to be treated if the same thing were happening to you. It can feel like trying to keep your head above water while drowning in the ocean during a storm. You are continually blasted with symptoms, tossed around violently, exhausted to the point of going under, and so desperate for someone to reach out their hand and pull you onto a boat. While you are frantically searching for a lifesaver, the last thing you want is to hear someone shouting unhelpful advice or hurtful opinions from shore. Offhanded comments, no matter how insignificant they seem, can fester. "You'll be fine. Stop being so lazy. You're too young to have that. Everyone gets tired..." *Whiner. Burden. Inadequate. Exaggerating. Useless.* Guilt (Day 10) is often self-inflicted, but when the people closest to you contribute to your feelings of self-blame—knowingly or unknowingly—it makes those feelings become an even heavier burden.

Believe them. You cannot truly support someone if you doubt them. Do not look at their good days as "proof" that they are lying about the bad ones (Day 23). Listen with the intent of understanding.

Learn more about their condition and symptoms. You do not need to become an expert, but an internet search or two can give you a good overview without costing you much time or effort. Or just ask them. Knowing the basics can help you start to understand what life is like for them. This can also help you recognize specific ways to offer support. Try using their language. "Do you have enough spoons (Day 8) for that today?"

Accept their limitations, let go of expectations, and be flexible. Allow for frequent breaks during an activity. Work with their dietary restrictions and be kind—those are not fun for anyone. Roll with the ups and downs. Understand that they might need to cancel plans without much warning. Do not expect them to always be available or to commit to social events. Forgive when these things are inconvenient.

Show interest. Go with them to a doctor's appointment. Exercise together. Join them for awareness events. Be a part of their journey. It will help them to feel less lonely. Remember that their condition is most likely for life and over time some of their support may have faded away.

If you do not live with chronic illness, do not always attempt to make comparisons to your own experiences. For example, assuming that you understand chronic fatigue (Day 12) because you have been really tired before, will likely make your loved one feel dismissed and even more alone (Day 18). You can show empathy without saying, "I know just how you feel."

Let them rest. It is so important and sometimes it is all they need in the moment.

Offer specific assistance instead of advice. It can be hard to ask for help, even when someone says, "Let me know if you need anything." Chronic pain sufferers often need help with a hundred little things and a statement like that can be overwhelming. *Did they really mean it or were they just trying to be nice? Should I actually ask? Will they think it's too much? Maybe they won't want to do that, but will agree out of a sense of obligation.* So offer specific assistance like picking up their prescriptions, making a meal, watching their kids so they can nap, doing their dishes, running an errand, driving them to an appointment, or many other things. You know them best. Every chronic illness is different and every person will have individual needs—even two people with the same condition might need different support. Think of a few clear-cut ways you can help, offer to do them, and most importantly, follow through.

It is okay if you cannot physically help. The best support you can give is continued love, understanding, compassion, and empathy. These go a long way. You can be an outlet for them to vent, brainstorm with, or just process their feelings. Be an active listener and help them know that they are not alone. It is easy to become overwhelmed by negative feelings. Chronic pain can make the sufferer feel isolated (Day 18), frustrated, guilty (Day 10), and depressed (Day 20). Their outlook may be shrouded in darkness, but you can help them feel hopeful and loved.

Now, it is important to mention that support is not only the obligation of others; the patients themselves bear some responsibility. Whether things are rapidly changing or you feel like you are stuck in a rut, it is helpful to connect with a community and many areas have local groups. Chances are you can find at least one other person who is going through similar things. And the more you open up, the more you will discover that you are not the only one. The wisdom and empathy of people who have been there and truly understand is priceless.

Use online support groups and social media not just for advice, but for connecting with people and being a part of something bigger. However, while online groups can definitely be an invaluable resource, they can also be harmful and soul-crushing. Be selective—some are drama-filled, stressful, and exhausting. Take a step back if you need to. It is not helpful to continually witness fighting and bullying or to be constantly reminded about the horrors of your condition. It is a big and important part of your life, but it is not your entire life. These groups can consume you and increase your stress level if you let them.

Ask for help. That seems so simple, but it can actually be incredibly difficult. It is embarrassing, especially if you have low self-esteem. Although, if you have high self-esteem, pride can get in the way because you do not want to be seen as weak. It is in our nature to want to do everything ourselves and not be a burden. Let people know what is going on. If someone genuinely offers to help—and you need it—then accept it. They will likely stop offering if you continually turn them down. Allow people who care about you to support you. While chronic illness can definitely be a burden, you are not. You are a valuable human being, so ask for help when you need it and accept it when it is offered.

Allow yourself to be vulnerable and honest. Vulnerability is not a weakness. It actually requires a great deal of strength. Sometimes people put up walls as a defense mechanism, thinking that it will protect them from getting hurt. But in reality, their protective shell also blocks out love and support from others. You have no control over how people will respond—good or bad. That is what makes it scary and risky, but that is also where strength and courage come in. It may feel easier and safer to just stay silent, but there is no long-term benefit to that. Nobody will ever know what you are going through or be able to help appropriately if you keep all that information to yourself. And you will eventually end up cutting yourself off from those who care about you.

Breaking your silence opens up the opportunity for support and compassion to become a part of your life. You do not need to give every detail of your journey all at once. After all, you did not learn everything in one overwhelming sitting—it came slowly over multiple appointments and doctors, countless hours of research, diagnosis after diagnosis, and other ways over time. Start small and allow people to process what they have heard. This gives you a chance to feel out how it is going and also gives your friends and family time to absorb the information. You might just find that this is the transformative step both you and your loved ones needed.

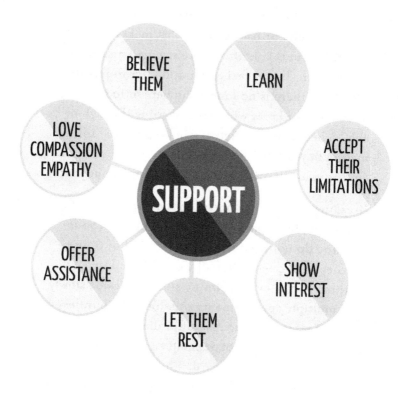

DAY 30:
Final Thoughts

It is not fun to be sick or in pain. Many chronic illness patients used to be active and social, but now they desperately search for answers and treatments in order to get back a sliver of what once was. It takes a lot of effort to manage the overwhelming symptoms.

Education is the first step to reducing pain. This can be more difficult than it sounds when some medical professionals are less than helpful (Day 13), and misinformation and extraordinary claims often fill internet search results. Gaining control of symptoms depends on each person's ability to gather information, find knowledgeable doctors who are willing to listen, and lean on supportive friends and family (Day 29). However, many healthy people lack understanding (Day 6), and as a result, sufferers often struggle to find encouragement and hope (Day 20). Because of inaccurate diagnoses, gaps in knowledge, and cultural stigmas (Day 7), treatment for many patients is inadequate at best and harmful at worst. A transformation in how people view chronic conditions is needed.

In order for change to truly happen, medical professionals need better ways of evaluating patients and sharing new information and treatments, and the general public needs to gain understanding. This will require a cultural shift in the way pain is both perceived and managed. The world is facing a pain crisis and it is time we address it.

People living with a chronic illness have to be self-disciplined in order to get enough rest, avoid trigger foods, take their medications, and dodge as many flare-ups as possible. It is understandable that sometimes you just want to feel normal. So you eat some ice cream or stay up too late, knowing that you will pay for it later (Days 8 and 27). The obstacles and hardships will always be there waiting for you like unwanted passengers who refuse to get out of your car. Despite struggling with guilt (Day 10), grief, isolation (Day 18), and debilitating symptoms, you push on because this is your life. It is a daily battle to be able to understand your own body and do things that others take for granted.

On the other hand, it can also foster surprising personal strengths, like empathy and the ability to persevere. Living with a chronic illness is a difficult way to develop these qualities, but you can either focus on your pain and let it control you, or you can choose to learn from it and grow despite your condition. It can help you find an inner strength that you never knew you had. Once you learn how to deal with the adversity, you gain more confidence in yourself and your good days become better.

I used to do half marathons, until my joints loudly informed me that that part of my life was over. However, during each race, I was always in pain and ready to quit by mile 10. I would wonder why I was even doing it and tell myself that this was the last one, never again. For the next couple of days, it was hard to get out of bed and it hurt to walk. And then after about a week, I was ready to sign up to do it all over again. Why?

I loved that it was something that my husband and I did together. I love the comradery and support of the running community—it is unparalleled. And the medal at the finish line was nice too. But the real high came from a sense of accomplishment, knowing that I was capable of making it through the pain, exhaustion, and negative thoughts. Adversity is unavoidable in life. At some point, everyone hits their own "mile-10 wall." For someone with a chronic illness, that might happen daily. But if you keep going, one breath at a time, you will have better days. We each have personal challenges, and they will most certainly change over time. So run your own race with patience and perseverance. Sometimes your goal will be mile 13.1 and other times it may only be a quarter of a mile. But if you chase after everyone who passes you, you will either burn out or end up off course.

When my son was young, I bought a rock tumbler because he was obsessed with rocks. According to the directions, the process was going to take a long time. Because that was not going to discourage us, we put everything into the barrel and started it up. It was incredibly loud. Trying to muffle the sound, we kept it in the downstairs bathroom, closed the door, and then waited. Days went by. The clanking got on my nerves and my son completely lost interest. About a week later, we gave up. That cold, muddy water and annoying thumping were working to make something beautiful, but we did not endure.

Life with a chronic illness can feel like that—endlessly tumbling in the dark and muck. Months, years, or decades go by and nothing seems to get better. We may even start to question our purpose and lose hope. But if we give up, we will never see the ugliness transform into something new. All that friction and grit does not take away our beauty; it actually reveals it. When we let them, our trials build strength and character. If you feel trapped, remember that all this tumbling is polishing you. Keep going and you will be left with something extraordinary.

I hope that everyone has learned something from this book. For healthy people, I hope that when someone with a chronic illness comes into your life, you will now be able to understand them a little better and are more aware that there is no one-size-fits-all for these conditions. For those who suffer with a chronic ailment, I hope that knowing the prevalence will help you open up, not feel so alone, and find the support you need. And I hope that we all get to a point where our world recognizes invisible illnesses and accepts the unique and valuable people who live with the symptoms every day.

Endnotes

1 Institute of Medicine. Relieving Pain in America: A Blueprint for Transforming Prevention, Care, Education, and Research. Washington, DC: National Academies Press; 2011.

2 National Center for Complementary and Integrative Health. Americans Spent $30.2 Billion Out-Of-Pocket on Complementary Health Approaches. https://www.nccih.nih.gov/news/press-releases/americans-spent-302-billion-outofpocket-on-complementary-health-approaches. 22 June 2016.

3 World Health Organization. Integrated chronic disease prevention and control. https://www.who.int/chp/about/integrated_cd/en/.

4 The Spoon Theory. Christine Miserandino. 2021. https://butyoudontlooksick.com/articles/written-by-christine/the-spoon-theory/.

5 Institute of Medicine. Relieving Pain in America: A Blueprint for Transforming Prevention, Care, Education, and Research. Washington, DC: National Academies Press; 2011.

6 The American Academy Of Pain Medicine. AAPM Facts and Figures on Pain. http://accurateclinic.com/wp-content/uploads/2016/04/AAPM-Facts-and-Figures-on-Pain-2011.pdf. 2011.

7 Partnership to Fight Chronic Disease. The Growing Crisis of Chronic Disease in the United States. http://www.fightchronicdisease.org/sites/default/files/docs/GrowingCrisisofChronicDiseaseintheUSfactsheet_81009.pdf.

8 Anna Zajacova, Hanna Grol-Prokopczyk, and Zachary Zimmer. Pain Trends Among American Adults, 2002–2018:

Patterns, Disparities, and Correlates. DOI 10.1215/00703370-8977691. 19 February 2021.

9 Mark H. Pitcher, Michael Von Korff, M. Catherine Bushnell, Linda Porter. Prevalence and Profile of High-Impact Chronic Pain in the United States. The Journal of Pain. DOI:https://doi.org/10.1016/j.jpain.2018.07.006. 07 August 2018.

10 Salynn Boyles. Cancer Risk Double for Women Smokers. 11 July 11 2006.

11 Hye-Kyung Jung. Is There True Gender Difference of Irritable Bowel Syndrome in Asia?. doi: 10.5056/jnm.2011.17.2.206. 27 April 2011.

12 Kristine Goodwin. National Conference of State Legislatures. Improving Women's Health State Policy Options. https://www.ncsl.org/Portals/1/Documents/Health/WHchecklist12-15.pdf. December 2015.

13 Institute of Medicine. Relieving Pain in America: A Blueprint for

Transforming Prevention, Care, Education, and Research. Washington, DC: National Academies Press; 2011.

14 The American Academy Of Pain Medicine. AAPM Facts and Figures on Pain. http://accurateclinic.com/wp-content/uploads/2016/04/AAPM-Facts-and-Figures-on-Pain-2011.pdf. 2011.

15 American Psychological Association. Gender and Stress. https://www.apa.org/news/press/releases/stress/2010/gender-stress. 2012

16 Affiliated Urologists. Why Women Get UTI's More Than Men. https://www.affiliatedurologists.com/blog/why-women-get-uti-s-more-than-men.

17 Keira J. A. Johnston , Joey Ward, Pradipta R. Ray, Mark J. Adams, Andrew M. McIntosh, Blair H. Smith, Rona J. Strawbridge, Theodore J. Price, Daniel J. Smith, Barbara I. Nicholl, Mark E. S. Bailey. Sex-stratified genome-wide association study of multisite chronic pain in UK Biobank. https://doi.org/10.1371/journal.pgen.1009428. 8 April 2021.

18 Institute of Medicine. Relieving Pain in America: A Blueprint for Transforming Prevention, Care, Education, and Research. Washington, DC: National Academies Press; 2011.

19 Dysautonomia International. Diagnostic Delay in POTS. https://www.dysautonomiainternational.org/page.php?ID=184#:~:text=The%20average%20diagnostic%20delay%20for,receive%20POTS%20related%20medical%20care.

20 National Resource Center on Lupus. Lupus facts and statistics. https://www.lupus.org/resources/lupus-facts-and-statistics#:~:text=On%20average%2C%20it%20takes%20nearly%20six%20years%20for,people%20with%20lupus%20surveyed%20report%20being%20incorrectly%20diagnosed. 6 October 2016.

21 Vishalli Ghai, Haider Jan, Fevzi Shakir, Pat Haines, Andrew Kent. Diagnostic delay for superficial and deep endometriosis in the United Kingdom. DOI: 10.1080/01443615.2019.1603217. 22 July 2019.

22 Jennifer Casarella, MD. WebMD. Dealing With Chronic Illnesses and Depression. https://www.webmd.com/depression/guide/chronic-illnesses-depression. 27 September 2020.

23 Table 19. Leading causes of death and numbers of deaths, by sex, race, and Hispanic origin: United States,

1980 and 2016. https://www.cdc.gov/nchs/data/hus/2017/019.pdf. 2017

24 L S Hitchcock, B R Ferrell, M McCaffery. National Library of Medicine. The experience of chronic nonmalignant pain. DOI: 10.1016/0885-3924(94)90190-2. 9 July 1994.

25 The American Academy Of Pain Medicine. AAPM Facts and Figures on

Pain. http://accurateclinic.com/wp-content/uploads/2016/04/AAPM-Facts-and-Figures-on-Pain-2011.pdf. 2011.

26 David W. Baker. The Joint Commission's Pain Standards: Origins and Evolution. Oakbrook Terrace, IL. 5 May 2017.

27 National Center for Drug Abuse Statistics. Opioid Epidemic: Addiction Statistics. https://drugabusestatistics.org/opioid-epidemic/#:~:text=Opioid%20Prescription%20Dispense%20Rates%20%20%20%20Year,%20%2079.5%20%2010%20more%20rows%20. 2019

28 Kevin E Vowles , Mindy L McEntee, Peter Siyahhan Julnes, Tessa Frohe, John P Ney, David N van der Goes. National Library of Medicine. Rates of opioid misuse, abuse, and addiction in chronic pain: a systematic review and data synthesis. DOI: 10.1097/01.j.pain.0000460357.01998.f1. April 2015.

30 DAYS
to UNDERSTANDING
AUTISM

CASEY CHAFFEY

Whether you are a novice or a veteran, navigating the overwhelming amount of information about autism can be daunting.

There is no shortage of books, articles, research, opinions, and misinformation. Autism spectrum disorder is one condition with common features that can manifest in diverse ways.

This book aims to be an easy and informal read while wading through a wide range of topics, including the following:

- ❊ *Communication and Executive Function*
- ❊ *Sensory Processing and Stimming*
- ❊ *Prevalence and Detection*
- ❊ *Depression and Learning Difficulties*
- ❊ *Studies, Statistics, and so much more*

---

30 Days to Understanding Autism can be read all at once, used as a reference guide, or simply be a place to turn for daily information and support.

Made in the USA
Middletown, DE
15 February 2022

61211284R00076